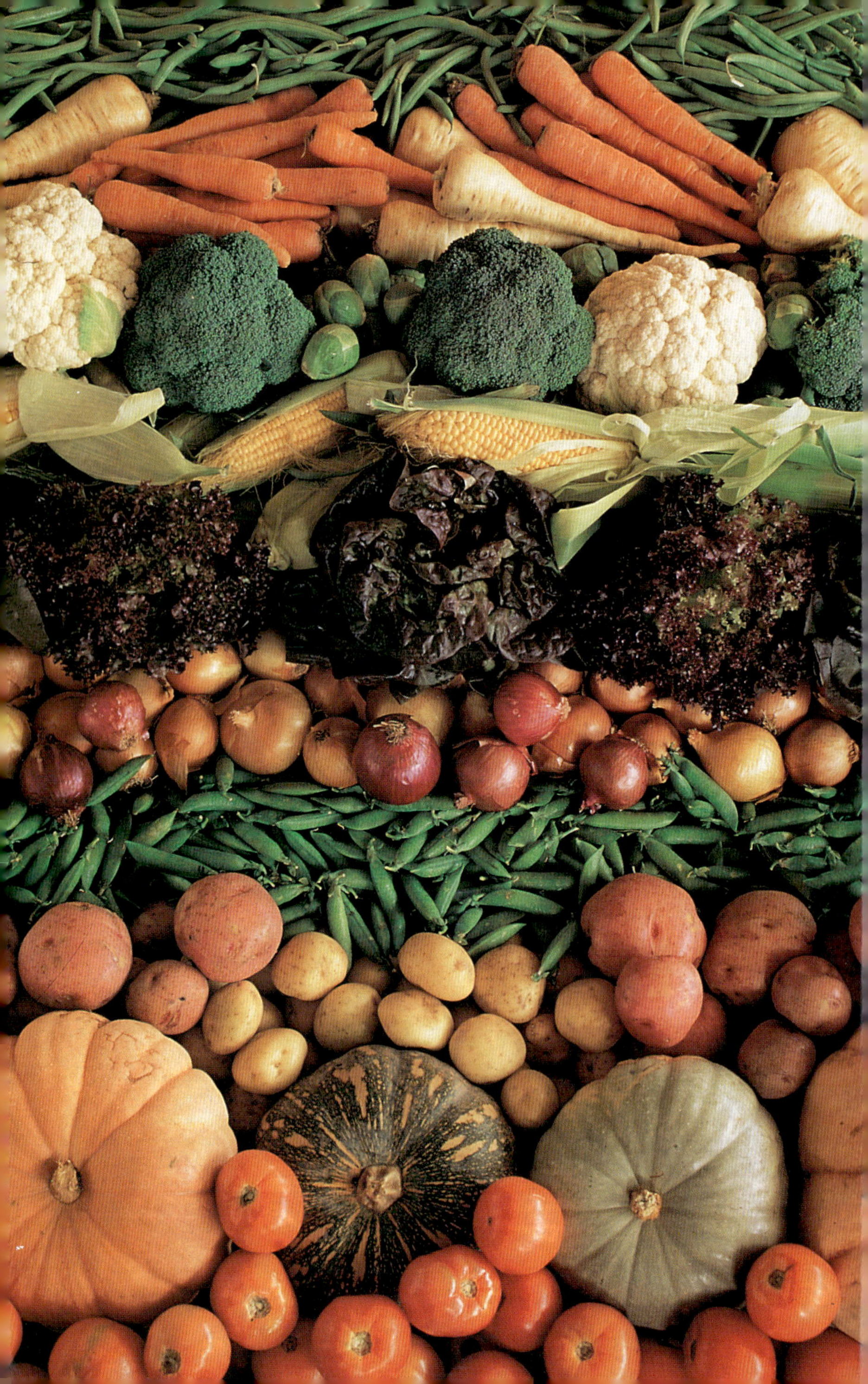

# Jackie French's

# TOP 10 Vegetables

Aird Books
MELBOURNE

Aird Books Pty Ltd
PO Box 122
Flemington, Victoria 3031



National Library of Australia
Cataloguing-in-publication data

French, Jackie.
Jackie French's top 10 vegetables.

ISBN 0 947214 38 0.

1. Vegetable gardening. 2. Cookery (Vegetables).
I. Title: Top ten vegetables.

635



Cover design and illustration by Helen Semmler
Photograph frontispiece by Virginia Wallace-Crabbe
Author photograph on backcover by Bryan Sullivan
Typeset in-house by Aird Books
Printed by Australian Print Group, Maryborough, Victoria

# contents

# *introduction*

This book is about the 10 most popular vegetables. Well, yes – but which? I love parsnips. My husband won't touch them . . . and refuses to admit there may be other parsnip lovers in this world. But then, he thinks no meal is complete without potatoes . . . and I prefer rice to spuds!

So who gets to decide which are the best?

According to our friendly local store, the 10 most popular vegetables (fresh or frozen) are potatoes, onions, tomatoes, lettuce, carrots, peas and beans, broccoli, pumpkin and corn.

According to a limited and not entirely random survey of radio listeners, friends and relatives (most of whom are vegie lovers) the 10 most popular vegetables are potatoes, carrots, tomatoes, lettuce, peas and beans, broccoli, pumpkin, corn and onions.

According to the Australian Bureau of Statistics, the most widely grown vegetables are potatoes, onions, tomatoes, lettuce, carrots, cauliflower (including other brassicas like broccoli, brussels sprouts and cabbages), pumpkin, corn and celery, followed by peas and beans – but most peas and beans eaten in Australia are frozen or otherwise processed – and a large proportion of these are imported.

So I've bumped beans and peas into the list . . . and there you have it: a book about (probably) the best loved, most eaten, most cooked and most appreciated veg!

All are infinitely better picked fresh: sweeter, crisper, crunchier and with more of the subtle flavours that get lost in storage, refrigeration, sorting, processing and packing. All are easy to grow, cheap and fun. I hope you enjoy them.

## *WHY GROW YOUR OWN?*

Because it's fun. Because unless you grow your own you won't taste vegetables as they really are: sweet, with texture and flavours lost a few hours (at most) after picking – the subtle tastes of sun and soil.

You can grow your own to save money: two lettuces a week will cost you about $80 a year. But if you grow your own lettuces you'll eat *many* more than two a week. You can grow your own to tempt yourself to eat more vegies. They are good for your health – and that's not counting the extra exercise, relaxation and deep satisfaction that goes with gardening.

You can grow your own because you remember your grand-parents with their fingers in the soil; because you dream of self-sufficiency; and because you want a healthy hobby and you are bored with bowls or jogging.

There are other reasons.

We need to learn to become growers, not destroyers; to learn that we are part of nature, subject to rain and storm and hail and drought. It's hard to insulate yourself from nature in a garden.

Yes, there are some gardeners who delight in producing the earliest tomatoes, whose gardens are so neat you feel terrified to tread on the scissored grass or pick a flower . . .

Most gardeners grow for the sheer love of it. Gardening – and growing our own – is part of our heritage of being human. It is one of my greatest joys.

### *Basic gardening*

For more information on basic – or eccentric – gardening methods, pest and weed control and companion planting, see the range of titles at the end of this book.

## *WHAT YOUR VEGIES NEED*

### *Soil*

If you don't have any soil – just shale or clay instead – don't panic. You can buy compost, soil or potting mix, or make an above-ground garden with hay, weeds, leaves and so on, and make your own soil.

### *Sunlight*

While many vegetables will grow in semi-shade, as a rule of thumb the vegie garden needs *at least* three hours of direct sunlight a day.

### *Water*

Vegies need less water if they are well mulched. On a hot day, sprinklers lose 90 per cent of their water to evaporation. Hose *under* the mulch instead – or install a dripper system.

### *Food*

If you keep harvesting your vegies without putting food back, your plants will slowly starve – and so will you if you are relying on those vegetables. Consult the relevant entry for each plant's food needs.

## *HOW TO START A GARDEN BED*

### *The dig-and-break-your-back method*

Dig deeply once; leave for three weeks for weeds to germinate; dig again, making sure you haul out all weed bits.

Now visit your chiropractor for back restoration.

Digging destroys soil structure, kills earthworms and other soil life – including nitrogen-fixing bacteria – and isn't necessary.

### *Above-ground beds*

Don't bother about newspaper – it can create an impenetrable layer between the soil and the mulch.

Pile old leaves or hay or dry weeds half-way up to your knees. Top with a finger depth of compost, potting mix or very good soil. Plant at once. Feed with liquid manure or fertiliser till the plants are established and the leaves, etc. are broken down – about one month.

### *Weed mat gardens*

Spread weed mat over weeds or grass. Weigh it down so it doesn't blow away. Cut holes, spoon out grass, weeds, sand and soil; plant seedlings. Water well – and feed well for at least a month till the grass and weeds below have broken down and passed their nutrients back into the soil.

### *WEEDS*

Get rid of weeds by:

- Piling mulch on top of them (best method).
- Pouring boiling water on them. (*Note*: be careful of plant roots).

**What to do with weeds**

Put down newspaper and pile the weeds on top – they make great mulch around the garden or as a start to make a new garden bed.

### *PESTS*

See individual entries. See also *The Wilderness Garden; Jackie French's Guide to Companion Planting;* and *Natural Control of Garden Pests. You* don't actually need to get rid of pests – or even feed your garden. Your garden should do it all by itself. These books will tell you how.

### *FEEDING YOUR GARDEN*

There are hundreds of ways to feed your garden. (See *Soil Food – 1372 ways to feed your garden*, Aird Books, 1995.) They include green manuring, growing 'nitrogen fixing' crops to add fertility to your soil, keeping chooks and other small animals, making compost in heaps or with earthworms. But if you just want a fertiliser to add to your soil, try

- Hen manure, either pelletised like Dynamic Lifter or home-grown (and at least six months old).
- Blood and bone
- Seaweed fertilisers
- Good mulches like lucerne hay (from some garden centres and stock and station agents) or lawn clippings (make sure they are dry, or they may heat up and burn your plants).
- Home-made compost
- Home-grown urine (your own doesn't smell as bad as other

people's) diluted with ten times the amount of water. Don't use this more than three times a year in any spot or you may raise the salt level – and be mindful of other people's sensitivities. Keep it away from, say, the lettuce – the base of a corn plant or tomato bush is probably more acceptable, particularly if no one knows about it.

- Home-made liquid manure: soak hen manure or other manures or seaweed or grass clippings or compost in water till it turns pale brown. Use every day on plants that need lots of feeding like corn and lettuce. The sludge at the bottom can be used too.

Liquid manure is infinitely variable. I add comfrey, chamomile, horseradish leaves and nettles to help disease resistance. Make sure you keep a lid on the bucket though to keep out mozzies, cats and dogs.

# *beans*

*(Beans) . . . move the belly, provoke urine, enlarge the breast that is straightened with shortness of breath, engender sperm, and incite to venery . . .*
NICHOLAS CULPEPPER

***If you can grow one sort of*** bean, ***you can grow other beans:*** bush beans, butter beans, climbing beans, perennial beans, red kidney beans, scarlet runner beans ***and*** soy beans.

### *ROOTS*

Beans were first cultivated in Peru about 6000 years ago. They were a staple food of the Aztecs, who didn't keep domestic animals. The conquistadors brought beans back to Spain, as well as the perennial bean or scarlet runner, which they brought back for its flowers, not realising the bean seed was also good to eat. (Broad beans were well-known in ancient Europe and when ancient sources mention beans that's what they refer to.)

Since the conquistadors sailed back in (probably gaseous) triumph, beans have become a staple in most parts of the world, either whole or dried or made into beancurd, or the fermented beancurd tempee, not to mention soy sauce, bean jelly and an enormous number of other bean products.

### *MEDICINAL BEANS*

Culpepper wasn't alone in thinking beans 'incite to venery'. The followers of Pythagoras were not allowed to eat beans, possibly for that reason, but also because it was believed that humans souls could return as beans. Bean lovers however shouldn't panic and think they may be driven mad with lust. Pythagoras and Culpepper probably referred to broad beans.

A diet high in bean curd has been associated with lower breast cancer rates, and other cancers. This may be because the fat intake is reduced when you swap to bean protein, but also because of possible impacts on hormonal levels. It is also possible that eating large (very large) quantities of beans may cause menstrual irregularities, lowered testosterone and fertility, especially in Western diets – but this is controversial and, I must emphasise, is based on studies of diets with a sugar bean component.

In one study by the University of Washington a half a cup of dried beans per day (cooked) reduced triglycerides by 17 per cent; half a cup of cooked beans a day may lower cholesterol by an average of 10 per cent. Swapping meat for bean curd will reduce the risk of kidney and gallstones. Beans help regulate blood sugar levels.

Beans are high in the trace element manganese and may help reduce bone loss with osteoporosis.

Beans are also provokers of flatulence extraordinaire, but if you eat a lot your gut gradually gets (almost) used to them, at least partially solving the problem.

## *BEAN VARIETIES*

There is a multitude of choice with beans – far more than you would expect from the choice at the supermarket.

Beans are either climbing (needing a trellis or room to hang down) or dwarf; either green or yellow or red fleshed with seeds either creamy, spotted, brown or purple; for use either fresh or dried; and either annual or perennial.

As I mentioned, I prefer climbing beans – you get more beans in a smaller space and climbing beans also seem more resistant to beanfly. They don't need weeding once they've started to clamber up their trellis or pole. You also don't have to bend down to find the beans for dinner – or stick your hands in reach of snakes. We also grow two sorts of perennial beans.

Apart from that, we tend to grow a good variety of beans – and colours of beans – always Purple Kings just for fun (though the taste and texture probably isn't as good as green or yellow beans and they are also more prone to rust) and yellow beans as well as green.

***Bush beans***

*Slenderette* A good stringless bean with slim pods; you get at least three good pickings; a good tasting bean.

*Windsor long pod* These are long beans (25 cm), and a very popular variety – good for 'best bean' competitions at local shows.

. . . and many others.

***Butter beans***

These are yellow, slightly sweeter and more tender than green beans and need slightly more warmth.

*Sylvan gold* Produces prolific crops and is also good shelled.

*Mammoth golden cluster* This is a climbing butter bean, with enormous clusters of slightly flattened beans. The beans can grow quite large, but get tough and need careful stringing – they are best eaten small and stringless.

. . . and many others.

***Climbing beans***

*Purple king* Watch for rust, and don't panic – the purple turns green when they're cooked.

*Blue lake* Stringless, with excellent flavour and a heavy crop – good in cooler areas.

*Epicure* Stringless when young, with good flavour.

*Westralia* A rust resistant, strong grower for hot and humid areas.

. . . and many others.

***Dried beans***

These include soy beans, bortolotti and red kidney beans – but most beans are good dried. See under 'Using your bean crop', p. 16.

***Perennial beans***

These are short lived perennials – though if you keep them mulched they'll survive for decades. There are at least three varieties – one with a pure red flower – Scarlet Runner, Penny

Bean, Seven Year Bean – one with a red and white flower, 'Painted Lady', and White Dutch with a white flower. All three beans have slightly different patterns on the bean. There is probably at least one more cultivar – we bought our Scarlet Runner beans from three sources and all are somewhat different.

Make sure you mulch climbing beans. The roots get bigger every year, so that finally they grow above the soil level – and can be damaged by digging, heat and especially frost.

Perennial beans are climbers, with brilliant coloured flowers – incredibly lovely wandering over a trellis. They don't set beans in hot weather unless they are either well mulched or otherwise shaded. We grow comfrey along the trellis where we grow our perennial beans and this shades the roots, so we do get perennial beans in mid summer. But even in very hot areas, with unshaded roots, perennial beans give an excellent autumn crop – and good summer or late spring crops for those dull cloudy seasons when it seems other beans will never mature.

Perennial beans get large and tough as they get older. They are best picked small and young – or left to mature and then the beans inside the pod picked and cooked like peas (delicious) or left to dry on the vine. They can then be used in any of the ways you'd use dried beans.

'And the scarlet coloured beans, in regard of the glorious beauty of their colour, being set near a quickset hedge, will bravely adorn the same by climbing thereon, so they may be discerned a great way away, not without admiration of beholders at a distance. But they will go near to kill the quicksets by clothing them in scarlet.'

### *Snake bean*

Also known as the yard-long bean or asparagus bean (*Vigna sesquipedalis*), this is a hot climate perennial with metre-long beans on vines up to two metres high. It is excellent in tropical and subtropical cimates, though you can grow it as an annual in temperate climates, or even in cool climates against a warm, north-facing wall.

## *CULTIVATION*

### *Why you should grow your own*

Beans may be treated with diazinon or dimethoate for bean fly. Diazinon is extremely persistent, extremely harmful to birds, bees and fish, and remains a long time in the environment. If polluted with water during storage or handling diazinon can become extremely toxic. (I have suffered from diazinon poisoning.) It is suspected as a teratogen; also of causing miscarriages.

Dimethoate is systemic and moderately toxic. It is deadly to bees and a suspect carcinogen.

Beans may also be polluted with endosulphan – an organochlorine, toxic to birds, earthworms and with possible delayed effects on human health.

Beans may be treated with benomyl before and after harvest as a fungicide to control blight. It has been shown to be mutagenic in tests with bacteria. It also kills earthworms.

Beans may be sprayed with zineb or mancozeb to control rust.

### *Essential information*

Beans are frost-tender annuals.

Plant after frosts. Feed till they start to flower. Mulch beans up to the bottom leaves to promote root growth along the stem. Pick beans young before they get stringy, and to stimulate more bean flowers. Pick often to encourage more flowers.

Home-grown beans snap. Supermarket beans bend. If your beans bend rather than snap it's not good eating. Throw them away and buy some bean seeds.

### *Bean seed*

You can grow dried beans and lentils from the supermarket or health food store. Choose fresh looking lentils or dried beans – ones with no dust at the bottom of the packet. Soak them overnight and plant. I have done this with soy beans, chick peas, lima beans, red kidney beans, green and brown lentils – it doesn't work with dried peas though. These may be partly cooked before they are dried.

### *Sowing*

*Tropical areas* February to October.
*Subtropics* All year round, cover with hessian, old bags, etc. to protect them from occasional light frosts during winter.
*Temperate areas* September to February.
*Cool areas* October to January (or when soil temperature reaches 16 to 20°C).

### *Germination and yield*

*Temperature range* 10-24°C, but beans prefer temperatures of 16°C or higher.
*Time taken to germinate* 7 to 10 days.
*Time until your first bean* 8 to 10 weeks; will crop for between 2 and 6 weeks depending on the variety and weather conditions.
*Successions* Plant the next lot of beans when the first lot is flowering.
*Number of plants for a family of four* 3 to 5 one-metre rows of dwarf beans; 1 to 3 one-metre rows of climbing beans, with more beans planted when those are flowering. This should also give you some beans for drying.

### *Planting*

Sow beans about 2.5 cm deep, 5 cm apart or two beans seeds together 10 cm apart in rows or in a square, or interplanted with marigolds or other companions to ward off beanfly. Don't place artificial fertiliser or hen manure straight over the bean seed – young bean plants are susceptible to fertiliser burn. Mulch the young plants instead and feed on top of the mulch.

One alternative way of growing beans is to plant each bean in a wide depression. This is then filled with mulch as the bean grows and traps moisture in very dry areas. Not recommended in wet areas or seasons.

I prefer climbing beans – you get many more beans per square metre and less area to water and weed – in fact climbing beans will outgrow most weeds once they're knee high if (and this is a big if) they are well fed and watered.

### *Feeding beans*

Beans will produce more beans even in poor soil – but you get a much better crop if they are fed, especially after they start to flower – the added food will mean they crop for much longer. Compost is, of course, the best food for beans, but any fertiliser will do. If you are mulching your beans you'll find that the nutrients from the decaying mulch will feed your plants through flowering time. In this case just give the mulch a light dusting of fertiliser like hen manure or blood and bone when beans are young to help the mulch begin to decompose.

Don't just scatter dry fertiliser near beans – bean roots are very susceptible to burning and you may kill the nitrogen fixing bacteria associated with these roots. These may also be killed (or at least suppressed) with a surplus of nitrogen.

Beans that are fed better are less susceptible to leaf eating or sucking pests like bean fly. Beans will form more roots up the stem if you hill them – either with compost or soil – and of course the more roots a bean plant has the more nutrients it is able to take from the soil – I like to mulch my beans right up to the first or second row of leaves. This isn't quite as effective as hilling, unless it is a very good mulch like partially broken down lucerne and the bottom part quickly turns into soil around the base of the plant. I dust my beans with wood ash when they are small to add potash. (On the other hand beans will die or twist with excess potash – don't assume that if a little is good more is even better.)

Beans prefer a pH of between 5 and 6.5, but if well mulched will still grow well in much more acid soil.

### *Other ways to grow beans*

#### *Beans in bottles*

Cut off the bottom of a plastic bottle. Thrust the bottom into the soil – water it first if it's hard. Throw in some mulch, then a bean seed and cover with a bit of compost or potting mix.

The bean will germinate quickly in its own hot house. As it grows keep mulching – up to the top of the bottle then around the bottle.

The advantage of this method is that you don't have to prepare a bean bed at all – just plant them in the lawn. All you need are enough bottles and mulch. The beans grow fast and should be healthy.

### *Beans in the living room*

Beans are an attractive indoor plant, especially in winter. Twine climbing beans up a pole and keep them near a window – Purple Kings can look lovely.

### *Beans in hanging baskets*

These dangle delightfully – especially scarlet runners or Purple King.

### ***Games with climbing beans***

Climbing beans can be grown on a traditional trellis. They can also be grown up a pole or spread out on an old bicycle wheel placed on top of the pole or grown up a tripod of stakes tied at the top. You can also make a circle of old chicken wire and fill it with compost and grow beans all around the wire. There are endless ways you can experiment with growing climbing beans.

You might also tie a rope to a fence or trellis and weigh it with a rock or stake it down – then grow beans up the rope. I have stretched string from window to ground and run climbing beans up the rope. This gives fast and productive shade to hot windows.

## *COMPANION PLANTING FOR BEANS*

The more you mulch your beans the more roots they put out. I grow borage with my beans. The borage repels beanfly or bean mites and the fast growing and fast decaying leaves can be used as mulch.

Corn planted with beans tends to increase the range of predators eating the pests of both beans and corn. I let our climbing beans ramble up the corn stalks. The beans don't give quite as good a crop (corn is a growth suppressant) but on the other hand they flower and crop slightly earlier.

Plant your beans when the corn is half grown.

A large number of vegies going to seed and flowering will attract predators to eat the pests on your beans. Nasturtiums will repel aphids and beanfly, but only if the beans are taller than the nasturtiums – and if there are a lot of nasturtiums. One measly plant near your bean crop will have no effect whatsoever.

I have also grown beans up sunflowers, planting the beans two weeks after the sunflowers emerged. They were slightly more resistant to beanfly – but on the other hand, sunflowers do inhibit the growth of beans slightly.

Marigolds are said to repel aphids and beanfly. I have tried this in trial beds for three years. The marigolds appeared to have no effect whatsoever on the beanfly population, but they did inhibit the growth of the beans slightly – less crop for a shorter period.

Marigolds are overrated as an effective companion crop.

## *GROWING PAINS*

### *Curling beans*

Beans curl in cool weather. They will straighten as it gets hotter.

### *Rotting seed*

Bean seed rots in cold wet weather. For early plantings coat with salad oil first. Add a sprinkle of white pepper to discourage ants or dust with old powdered tea leaves.

### *Fungus diseases*

Brown patches on leaves of beans; rotting stems; beans stuck together with brown or white fungus patches.

Spray with bordeaux spray if the temperature is under 24°C; spray every two days with chamomile tea. Plants mulched with comfrey or compost are much more resistant and will grow new roots up their stems to increase nutrient uptake.

### *Red spider mite*

Slight webbing on foliage, dull rough leaves.

A good overhead watering should control red spider problems. Interplant with marigolds or nasturtiums or mustard to repel them. Use milk spray, pikelet spray, anise or coriander sprays. Mulch half way up the stem with well rotted hay, manure or compost. This will encourage new roots – and vigorously growing plants are more resistant to mites.

### *Bean fly*

Plants or leaves collapse, tunnelling in stems.

Spray with dilute clay spray or pikelet spray. Try traps of sticky boards painted yellow and covered in glue or motor oil; use garlic spray; dust with derris every three days; hill plants around the base to encourage new roots or mulch half way up the stem with well rotted hay, manure or compost. This will encourage new roots – and vigorously growing plants are more resistant to bean fly.

Climbing beans are more resistant to bean fly, in particular Purple Kings, and snake beans are relatively unaffected. In bad areas try growing beans in cooler weather. Bean fly is usually a problem of poor soil, especially soil that is deficient in potash. Grow a comfrey border and use the leaves as mulch to utilise the potash in your soil – or add a potash rich fertiliser or wood ash. After two or three year of fertilising with compost you should find the problem disappears. Plant masses of flowering umbelliferae like fennel and parsnips, as well as grevilleas, or encourage predators to control the problem naturally.

***Rust***

Orange yellow pustules on leaves; leaves may yellow and fall off. For treatment, see Fungus diseases.

## *FROM THE GARDEN TO THE TABLE*

***Picking your beans***

Pick beans when they are young, sweet and tender, before the seeds swell and you can see them bulging in the pod. This will also promote more flowers. They need to be picked about every second day – and at least twice a week.

Take care when picking them as the stems can be fragile. A gentle twist rather than a hard pull is best. You soon get the knack of it.

***Using your bean crop***

Use beans straight away if you can – the flavour and texture of very fresh beans is quite different from even 1-day-old ones, though beans do keep for weeks in the fridge.

*Fresh eating period* Roughly the frost-free period minus 12 weeks; well-mulched high climbers may crop even with light

frosts. Mulch them deeply to keep them fruiting longer. Plant another crop as soon as the first is flowering for continuous beans.
*Food value* This is 126 kj per 100 g, a small amount of vitamin C and minerals and fibre. Protein varies according to the variety but may be higher per weight than meat.
*Storage time* You can keep beans one to two weeks in the fridge. They can be frozen, but it's better to rely on a succession of peas, leeks and spinach when the beans are finished.
*Surplus* Any bean can be dried. The most common are red kidney beans and soy beans, as well as borlotti beans. I love dried scarlet runner beans. Leave them on the bush till the pods are dry, then uproot the whole plant and bash it against a wall so the beans fall out on old newspaper on the ground. Gather the beans and keep them dry, away from light.

*EATING BEANS LIKE PEAS*
If your beans get too big and tough to eat whole treat them like peas – push out the seeds and eat them fresh, boiled or steamed for about five minutes, by themselves or with a knob of butter or a squeeze of lemon juice or a little finely diced fried bacon – just toss the beans in the grease. (I know this sounds horrid, and your arteries will probably agree – but it tastes good.)

*STEWED DRIED BEANS*
Wash 500 g dried beans – don't soak them. Sauté an onion in half a cup of olive oil, add the beans and cook slowly till the beans have absorbed most of the oil. Add a litre of hot water, garlic and a sprig of mint. Don't add salt – you'll toughen the beans. Cover the pan and stew as slowly as you can till all the liquid is dissolved. Eat hot or cold with a drizzle of lemon juice.

*LEATHER BRITCHES*
Leather britches are an American term for dried green beans. Thread them together with a darning needle so they hang in a row strung out in the sunlight for a few days, taking them in at night. Store in glass jars when they snap instead of bend. Soak them before using them – at least overnight – then simmer all day before eating them. Leather britches can be tough and awful if the

beans were old when they were dried or satisfying and stodgy if the beans were young and tender to start with.

*SOY BEAN CURD*

Dry soy beans in the oven till they are crisp. Grind them to flour in a flour mill or with a mortar and pestle. Take two cups of soy flour and add eight cups of cold water. Leave for half an hour, stirring a couple of times. Transfer to a pot, bring to the boil, keep stirring or it will stick on the bottom. Take off the heat and add three tablespoons of lemon juice at once. Keep stirring. Cool (don't chill it in the fridge). Line a colander or sieve with cheese cloth or even a tea towel. Tip the mixture in and leave overnight.

Store bean curd in the fridge when it is set, covered with water.

*BEAN JELLY*

Put three cups of beans in a pan with a very little water. Cook till soft. Add more water as necessary. When the beans are cooked press them through a sieve so the juice is extracted. This will set by itself. Eat fresh, or keep in the fridge.

*BEANS WITH TOMATO*

Heat a frying pan. Throw in olive oil and a generous amount of chopped garlic and a little chopped onion (and a chopped red chilli too if you like chilli). Cook for ten seconds and add your beans – topped and tailed, whole or chopped. Stir fry as hot as possible till the beans turn bright green – not very long; then throw in a couple of peeled chopped tomatoes. Keep stirring till the tomatoes are hot and just starting to break up.

Serve hot or cold with lots of black pepper.

*COLD BEANS WITH OIL AND LEMON*

Steam beans till they turn bight green – a few minutes is enough for young beans; older beans need more cooking to tenderise. Take off the heat. Dress at once with two parts olive oil to one part lemon juice, with lots of chopped garlic and a little French mustard and salt and pepper to taste.

Serve warm or cold.

# *carrots*

*Carrots . . . should be rais'd in Ground naturally rich, but not too heavy . . .*

EVELYN, ACETARIA, *A Discorse of Salets*, 1699

***If you can grow*** carrots ***you can grow*** parsnips ***and*** beetroot.

## *ROOTS*

Like all vegetables, carrots used to grow wild – thin, pale purple roots that were gradually improved to long, pale yellow carrots then, quite recently, into the deep orange varieties we know today. Early carrots were quite bitter, tougher, thinner and probably went to seed sooner. Medieval herbalists preferred wild carrots to domestic ones – their medicinal properties were said to be greater.

The ancient Greeks called carrots *philon*, from *phio*, loving. They were supposed to be an aphrodisiac – whether because of their taste, their medicinal properties, or their phallic appearance I don't know. Carrots were also supposed to be soporific, which presumably would have negated their use in provoking amorousness. Nowadays, herbalists don't ascribe either aphrodisiac or soporific qualities to carrots . . . maybe they disappeared when carrots were domesticated.

British fighter pilots in World War II were fed large quantities of carrots. This might have accounted for the pilots' amorous reputation. It was also supposed to have made them see better in the dark. In reality, the pilots' accuracy at night was due to radar, not to carrots – it was just a ruse to flummox the enemy.

## *MEDICINAL CARROTS*

Raw carrots or carrot juice is said to inhibit a range of cancers, or help prevent them. Carrot seed tea (make sure they aren't treated with fungicide) is said to help digestion and stop flatulence. (Eating raw carrots though is a great way to get flatulent in the first place.) Eating one fresh carrot is said to help reduce the risk of heart attacks (even more than most other vegetables). Eating carrots every day will reduce your chances of having a stroke by over half according to a recent Harvard study – and the beta carotene and vitamin A will increase your chances of recovery after a stroke and you should have less neurological damage. Foods high in beta carotene like carrots may also help avert cancer of the lung and larynx. Carrots are also high in roughage – good for constipation.

## *CARROT VARIETIES*

*Note*: Most carrot varieties still aren't hybrids . . . but hybrids are gaining ground (pun intended).

Carrots are never sold by name in supermarkets, so most people don't realise that different varieties taste . . . well, different. The best tasting carrot isn't necessarily the deepest orange one – in fact, deep orange carrots may be bitter or insipid.

The first couple of years you grow carrots, grow several varieties. Mark the name of each. (I usually forget to mark my varieties till I've forgotten which went where – and then, when we get a fabulous carrot, I don't know what sort it is.) Work out which you like best and which suits your climate best (the two may not be the same) – then stick to two or three varieties a year with maybe one new one every year for interest.

*Note*: I *always* grow several varieties of carrots – the weather changes every year, so that one lot may go to seed if it is unseasonably hot or cloudy; or they may crack if it's wet; or just sit there and do nothing . . . Growing at least three sorts, you're sure of getting a year's supply of carrots.

***Baby carrots***

These can be any young carrots, or one of several varieties like 'Amsterdam forcing', bred to mature small and early. They are generally sweet, tender and good.

***Mini round paris market***

These are small, almost round carrots – fat and juicy and good for thin soils.

***Belgium white***

A white heirloom variety from Digger's Club with green shoulders; won't survive below –5°C.

***King west***

These are very red carrots – long, thick, sweet and fast growing.

***All seasons***

Virus resistant. This can be sown all year in mild areas; in cool areas though they won't grow much during winter – and of course, like all carrots, will go to seed in spring.

***Topweight***

As the name suggests – very large carrots. They can be massive – but not as sweet as most others. With 'Western red' they are probably the most popular carrots in Australia.

***Nantes***

These are wonderfully sweet, orange rather than red, and medium sized.

***Red hot hybrid***

This is a very uniform carrot – perfect for supermarkets: deep orange, resistant to running to seed and resistant to splitting in wet weather.

***Early horn***

Early maturing variety with short roots for shallow soils. A pale but reasonably well flavoured carrot

***Round french***
Small round carrots, good for growing in boxes or on stony soil, or if you want a quick crop in spring or before winter.

***Tom thumb***
Another round rooted carrot for poor soils; fast maturing – about 12 weeks.

***Western red***
One of the mammoths, dark and sweet and *big* – possibly Australia's most popular carrot.

***Amsterdam forcing***
A quick growing 'baby' carrot.
. . . and many others.

## *CULTIVATION*

***Why you should grow your own***
Carrots may be treated with fungicides for post harvest watery soft rot (*Sclerotinia scleratiorum*).

***Essential information***
Carrots are biennial. (They go to seed the spring after sowing.) Don't overfeed them or use fresh manures. Carrots prefer well-dug deep soil – but you can get a decent crop without either.

There is nothing like the crunch of a carrot. Carrots add sweetness and richness to stews and soups and salads, without adding too many calories. Like all home-grown veg, if you haven't tasted a well grown, home-grown carrot, you don't know what carrots can taste like – rich and sweet and subtle.

***Carrot seed***
Carrots go to seed the spring after they have been planted – unless poor growing conditions make them go to seed earlier. (After all, if you were in fear of life from flood or heat you'd probably want to propagate too.)

In very cold areas where carrots may rot in permanently frozen ground, lift them in autumn, cut off the tops and keep in a dry dark space. Replant in spring and wait for new tops to emerge.

Carrot flowers with a great umbrella-like white bloom made up of hundreds of tiny flowers, each of which will set into a seed. Insects love carrot flowers – especially many tiny wasps that may help clean up insect pests from your garden.

Carrots are insect pollinated, and if two or more varieties are flowering at once (which may not be likely unless there are other dedicated vegie growers nearby) they'll cross pollinate. Unless you are trying to keep a special variety, cross pollination may not matter – especially as most carrots are still open pollinated, not hybrids (see varieties).

I just leave my carrots to go to seed, and stake them in wet windy weather – or just hope that enough will stay upright to give me next year's seed – and, as you get about 120 g from one carrot head, there isn't much danger of not having enough.

If you want to collect all the seed, tie an old stocking around the head as it is maturing. I just pick off the seeds from the top umbrella for my own use (they are said to be the strongest) and let the others fall to the ground. This gives me self-sown carrots, most of which will go to seed before they make good bottoms, as they'll be sown too late in the year. But sometimes you may be lucky and get a self-sown beauty. Then let it go to seed too – and you'll have a variety you can leave to grow itself in your garden.

Carrot seed lasts about three years in an old envelope, kept in a dark dry place. Some old gardeners reckon that older seeds – three or four years old – are best. Most won't germinate – but those that do will be tough. Given that you get so much carrot seed when you save your own, this is worth trying.

### *Sowing*

In all but the coldest areas carrots can be grown all year round – though 'grown' is a bit of an overstatement, as carrots won't grow in cold weather – they'll just sit there until spring and go to seed as soon as the weather warms up. However, unless your ground freezes totally in winter you can sow one crop of carrots in spring, when the soil warms up (if you plant the carrots into cold soil they'll go to seed as soon as the weather warms up) and then more carrots till say January – if you need more – as more land becomes available as you finish say crops of peas or broad beans.

Be careful with very early carrots – they are more prone to virus diseases, and it may be best to use a hybrid virus resistant variety for the earliest planting.

Carrots are a good adaptable crop for most areas – so delicious that humans have bred types to crop under almost any conditions, including an almost total lack of soil – though to get those great, perfect, long monsters you need rich, friable, lovely, deep soil.

Carrots also give a good crop for a small space.

*Tropical areas* February to November.

*Subtropical areas* Year round. If your grass stops growing in winter regard yourself as temperate for the purposes of growing carrots.

*Temperate areas* January to March. (Sow only small, fast-maturing varieties from January on.)

*Cool areas* September to January.

### *Germination and yield*

*Temperature range* 7-25°C, but prefers at least 16°C. May not germinate well over 30°C – see Lettuce.

*Time for eedlings to emerge* 10 to 21 days, depending on the weather.

*Time till first picking* 12 to 20 weeks – if you are prepared to eat tiny carrots. You can keep picking till next spring.

*Number of sowings* Carrots only need to be sown once a year in most parts of Australia.

*Number needed for a family of four* 6 to 12 square metres will give you lots of carrots every day.

### *A year of carrots*

I plant all our carrots in spring. If space is tight, you can keep planting carrot seed till late summer. I like to grow several varieties, but my tastes vary from year to year. I suppose that means not one carrot variety is really outstanding – and that variation is fun.

Tiny carrots will be ready for thinning after about two months. Eat them small and sweet and leave room for the others to expand.

Carrots get sweeter through winter. In early spring, mulch the ground around your carrots well to keep it cold, so your carrots don't go to seed till the next lot are ready to thin.

Deeply dug or soft soil gives long straight roots. Our carrots wriggle because I don't dig. But they are still thick and sweet.

Don't be tempted to grow carrots too late in the year. No, the frost won't kill them – but all you'll get will be carrot tops, not carrot bottoms. The latest date for sowing carrots is Christmas in cold climates, February in temperate climates. In tropical climates sow carrots from February to November – avoid sowing in the wet, hot, humid months.

### *Planting*

Carrots prefer well-dug soil, finely cultivated so that there are no lumps to make the roots fork. If carrots can't force their roots into the soil they'll grow upwards instead, or turn bulbous or fork into several small tributaries – which makes peeling and cleaning difficult, though the carrots still taste as good.

If your soil is poor or shaley, above-ground beds are best, as the carrots get more 'legroom' before they strike the tough bits.

Smooth out the soil before you plant carrots, otherwise the seed may all wash together. It is *very* hard to sow carrot seed thinly and evenly – you often get great clumps, and usually too many carrots close together. Try mixing the carrot seed with dry sand, or even dry tea leaves (this keeps away ants as well).

Cover the carrot seed with the finest possible sprinkling of soil or compost – no great clumps that will smother it. Water often and lightly. If you water too hard you'll wash the seed away; and if you don't water, the thin layer of soil will dry out and kill your young carrot shoots.

### *Feeding carrots*

Carrots prefer slightly acid, humus rich soil. Heavy clay soils will stunt them. When boosted with high nitrogen fertilisers you tend to get all tops and no bottoms.

Like all root vegetables carrots do not do well with undecomposed organic matter – either hen manure or animal manure. It may cause them to rot or become otherwise diseased and prone to insect attack. They may also fork (though they will do this in hard or rocky soil too).

Carrots do best where the ground has been well manured for a previous crop like lettuce or celery. You can also grow carrots in a bed of compost on top of the undug soil, about a handspan deep. Scatter the seeds, well-mixed with sand to spread them thinly, then scatter a little more compost on top. Don't press down. The vigorous roots will penetrate the soil below. They may fork – but they'll still be fat and good. In dry times they may also grow above the soil. This above-ground carrot will be deep green and very slightly bitter as well as sweet.

If you have totally unprepared soil, dig the soil at least 30 cm deep and sprinkle on half a cup of blood and bone or old hen manure per square metre.

If your carrots have hairy roots they've been grown in soil that's too rich in nitrogen, or deficient in phosphorus. Pale carrots may have been grown in phosphorus-deficient soil – though some varieties are paler than others.

Carrots prefer a pH of between 5.5 and 6.5.

### *Keeping carrots weed free*

Many novice gardeners plant their carrots then forget about them – and the poor little seedlings are overwhelmed by weeds. Carrots need excellent weeding until they are mature. Then, if they're planted close together, they'll keep the weeds out themselves.

I like to cover my dug soil with clear plastic before sowing carrots. This encourages weeds to germinate. When you are ready to plant your carrots take off the plastic, 'scratch' the soil, then plant.

I also plant carrots where I have had a weed mat bed before. When you pull up the weed mat the ground is weed free below.

You can also let brassicas go to seed in spring (see Cauliflowers) – then, when you haul them out after they've gone to seed, the ground will be relatively weed free – and dug over by the roots of cabbage, broccoli, etc. I also use radishes as 'natural diggers'.

### *Other ways to grow carrots*

#### *Above-ground carrots*

It is a myth that carrots need deeply dug soil. Carrots will do their own digging – they may just bend a bit in the process. Above-ground garden beds are excellent for carrots.

Spread one sheet only of newspaper on the grass (don't use any more or you may end up with an impermeable layer of newspaper) and cover with a thin layer of potting mix; or no newspaper and a thick layer of compost (at least 10 cm). Sprinkle on the carrot seed. Scatter on a thin layer of straw or dried lawn clippings. Water every day till the seedlings appear as the thin layer of soil or compost will dry out quickly. The carrots will grow through the paper into the undug soil.

Don't thin carrots – just pull them up when they are finger sized, and the little ones next to them will have more room to grow. Carrots are best sown in spring for year-round eating, though they taste best after a frost. 'Red chantenay' seem to resist going to seed longest in spring.

*Carrots in a box*

This method is weed free – good for novice gardeners. Fill a styrofoam box with potting mix. Make sure it has holes in the bottom. Scatter carrot seed thinly, cover with a very fine scatter of more potting mix. Water gently every day. Thin out carrots as they grow and crunch the little ones.

You'll be surprised how many carrots will fit into a box. Good for every balcony, as long as it gets at least three hours of sunlight a day.

### *COMPANION PLANTING FOR CARROTS*

Carrot fly are repelled by onions, leeks and other alliums, and by strong herbs like rosemary, wormwood, sage and salsify.

For bad cases of carrot fly, sow carrot seed together with spring onion seed, or keep a permanent band of spring onions around your carrot bed. The onions need to be actively growing to be effective. (Try cutting off the tops, so more grow.) You need at least twice as many spring onions as carrots. Chives and other onions or leeks will do as well – but again, there must be a lot of them, actively growing.

Strongly scented tomato foliage will also repel carrot fly, so grow blocks (not rows) of tomatoes and carrots next to each other.

## *GROWING PAINS*

### *Poor germination*

Snails love carrot seedlings. Watch out for them. I throw in radish seed with our carrot seed – the vigorous radish seed breaks up the soil for the smaller carrots and helps keep snails away. Fresh home-grown carrot seed always performs better than bought seed – let at least two carrots go to seed, and tie a paper bag around the seed heads to catch the ripe seed as it falls.

Carrots germinate poorly if the soil lacks humus and forms a thin crust on top. Again, try sowing carrot and radish seed together. The radishes will emerge first and break up the soil. Or sprinkle a thin layer of lawn clippings or sawdust with your seed or cover with hessian till the seeds sprout. If ants are a problem add some white pepper to the carrot seed.

### *Cracked carrots*

Carrots crack with too much rain or uneven watering. Plant them in a well drained spot and mulch so they don't dry out. Alternating very wet and very dry soil is a sure recipe for cracking. This can also be due to using artificial or strong high-nitrogen fertilisers like hen manure. Don't. Carrots don't like them.

### *Pink rot*

This is found in wet, badly drained soils. Improve drainage or raise the beds. In wet conditions carrots grown with a no-dig method do better than those in deeply dug soil.

### *Nematodes, root eelworm*

This shows as deformed, lumpy carrots with small swellings on the top. Try a preliminary crop of mustard. Keep up levels of organic matter. Mulch. Compost will inhibit nematodes and a good layer of steadily decomposing mulch, with a scatter of high-nitrogen material like old hen manure or urine on top is the best control. As a temporary measure, use molasses in ten parts water to dehydrate them. In bad cases leave ground fallow for a month – without any cover at all, including weeds. A rigorous crop rotation will keep down nematode numbers to non pest levels.

***Carrot aphid***

These small, green insects in the foliage congregate on the underside of the carrot tops. Try a vigorous hosing. As a last resort use marigold or pyrethrum spray. Marigolds or nasturtiums grown in between and around the crop may deter them as well as a nearby hedge of clipped wormwood.

***Premature bolting***

These carrots may lack nitrogen or phosphorus, in which case you should feed them with mulch or compost – but most likely you have sown them too late in autumn or too early in spring. While carrots survive most frosts, they will go to seed in any warm weather after a cold spell. Some varieties also tend to go to seed in very hot weather, or if grown in too much shade.

***Carrot fly larvae***

These burrow into the roots. They prefer straight rows. Sow carrots in blocks not rows. For bad cases sow carrot seed with spring onion seed and sow both together or keep a permanent band of spring onions round your bed. The onions must be actively growing to be effective, and must be in similar or greater numbers than the carrots. See also under companion planting.

***Bacterial soft rot***

Soft rot, which causes a soft smelly mess, is usually a post harvest problem, with damaged carrots stored in plastic or badly ventilated areas. If it occurs in the ground, the carrots have probably been damaged by weeding or digging. Mulch instead of weeding, or water first and pull instead of digging. Make sure the soil is well drained. Don't replant carrots where rot has been a problem for at least three years.

To prevent soft rot in storage, dry carrots in the sun after pulling. Keep in a well ventilated spot. If they must go into bags, use netting or paper, not plastic.

***Forked carrots***

Carrots may have been forced to fork by stones in the soil, though well fertilised carrots in compost rich soil, even if the soil below is hard as a rock, tend to grow up – and straight – if they can't grow down. Feed them better – add compost or good mulch. Carrots also fork when the soil is over-rich in nitrogen – grow them after a greedy crop such as lettuces or brassicas.

### *Pale carrots*

These may be lacking in phosphorus – add ground phosphorus or hen manure to your soil. They may also just be 'hungry' in poor soils. Also add potash for a good colour, avoid high-nitrogen fertilisers which may increase an imbalance of other nutrients; add lime to the soil to make nutrients more available in very acid soils.

### *Green tops on roots*

If a carrot is exposed to sunlight it turns green. Mulch well.

### *No roots*

Too much nitrogen, or else you planted too late or early in the year and the carrot is running to seed without rooting.

## *FROM THE GARDEN TO THE TABLE*

*Fresh eating period* All year from initial spring sowing.
*Storage time* Three months in fridge or cool cupboard; large quantities can be stored in newspaper. Carrots can be frozen, but I wouldn't bother – they get soggy and lose a lot of their flavour. If you are going to, dip them in boiling water for a second first, dry thoroughly then freeze as fast as possible – use an empty freezer and only put a few carrots in at a time. The faster they freeze the less squishy they'll be. If you make a lot of carrot cakes try grating the carrots first – they freeze a lot faster and you can fit more into a small space.

Take the tops off carrots if you are going to store them in a cupboard or in the fridge – they stay plump longer. (Yes, I know carrots look lovely with their ferny tops, but the root keeps feeding the leaves – and the carrot shrivels much faster.) I like to take the green shoulders off too – that also seems to help the carrots last better.

Keep carrots cool if you are transporting them, carrots shrivel in dry hot weather.

*Food value* 151 kj per 100 g. Rich in vitamin A, some vitamin C, potassium, calcium, phosphorus.

*Note*: If you really want to present a bunch of carrots, leaves and all, to a friend – and a bunch of leafy carrots is one of the glories of home-grown produce – stick the carrot roots in a bucket of water, so they stay plump. Don't keep them there longer than 24 hours – and be warned, this will also make them lose some of their vitamins.

***When to pick carrots***

Carrots can be picked as soon as they are big enough to bother with. I always eat the 'thinnings' – the ones I haul out so the rest can grow big. Remember though that carrots taste sweetest after the first frost – and are tenderest when young.

As soon as the soil warms up in spring carrots will prepare to go to seed. They become insipid, the centres will get tougher, till finally the leaves on top shoot up and the centre gets very tough indeed.

You can still use 'gone to seed' carrots. Just peel them, then slice or grate away the outside till you're left with the tough core. Peel away the outside tough bit and you'll have tender inside carrot left.

Or grate the whole lot to make dog biscuits.

*GONE-TO-SEED CARROT DOG BISCUITS*

Grate three large carrots. Add an equal weight of rolled oats or wheat germ. Moisten with an egg or two. Bake in a slow oven till crisp. Store in an airtight container.

***Dealing with a carrot surplus***

Carrots can be left in the ground until spring in most places. (If the soil freezes through winter dig them up before it does, cut the green leaves off, and store in a cool dark place.) If you have a surplus in spring, try dried carrots.

*DRIED CARROT*

Peel carrots – the skin may make the dried carrot bitter. Grate them; spread on alfoil in the sun or a cool oven. Dried carrots are rubbery when ready.

Add dried carrots to soups and stews to thicken and sweeten them. They reconstitute quickly.

### *Fresh carrot recipes*

Like all root vegetables, carrots are sweetest in winter, with a deep, rich colour. They can be eaten whole, dipped in mayonnaise or dressing, sliced into matchsticks or grated so finely they are almost liquid. (I'm munching a raw carrot as I write – I usually have carrot on and at the computer. A large crunch of carrot clears the brain.)

I usually peel carrots. The skin is often bitter, especially if there has been some check in the carrots' growth, or they have been badly stored.

#### *CARROT AND CORIANDER SALAD*

Peel carrots – carrot peel can be bitter – grate them, add an equal amount of well chopped coriander and dress with vinaigrette.

#### *CARROT AND BEETROOT WINTER SALAD*

Grate equal amounts of raw carrot and raw beetroot. Add some chopped parsley, and moisten with a very garlicky vinaigrette dressing.

This looks gorgeous – like a vampire's delight – and tastes excellent. Don't let the idea of raw beetroot put you off. And don't forget the garlic.

#### *GLAZED CARROTS*

This is good for insipid carrots. Just boil your carrots with not much water and a good glop of honey (not sugar). Boil till almost dry. The carrots will be sweet and even more richly coloured – and won't taste in the least honeyish unless you've overdone it with a strong variety like leatherwood.

#### *CARROT STICKS*

Chop your carrots into long thin sticks and tie in small bunches with a piece of parsley or fennel or a thin piece of red capsicum. Coat the tops and bottoms with a thick sauce – preferably one of the mayonnaises.

### *CARROT AND CHERVIL SOUP*

Simmer six grated carrots, six cups stock (chicken or good veg stock), one chopped onion and four chopped shallots for ten minutes. Whiz it all through the blender, or don't bother. Add three tablespoons of chopped chervil, reheat, then add a dash of cream and a little fresh chopped chervil on top.

### *CARROT GINGER BREAD*

125 g butter
100 g brown sugar
125 g self raising flour
2 eggs
1 dessertspoon treacle
2 teaspoons ground ginger
2 dessertspoons crystallised ginger, finely chopped
125 g carrots, grated
2 tablespoons ground almonds

Melt the butter, add the treacle and sugar, stir well. Take off the heat, stir in the eggs, then add the other ingredients. Moisten with a little milk if necessary.

Bake in a slow oven for an hour, or till a skewer comes out clean. (This will depend on the size of the cake tin.)

Leave uniced, or spread thinly with lemon icing when cold.

#### *Lemon icing*

Add a dash of lemon juice to icing sugar, with one tablespoon of butter for every cup of icing sugar. Don't add too much juice at once in case it gets too runny – just add more as necessary.

### *CARROT LEAVES*

These are edible, though often strong-tasting. Try a little carrot top chopped like celery in a mixed salad.

# *cauliflower*

*This I am sure, cabbages are extremely windy whether you take them as meat or medicine; yea, as windy meat as can be eaten, unless you eat bagpipes or bellows, and they are both seldom ate in our days . . .*
NICHOLAS CULPEPPER

***If you can grow*** Cauliflower ***you can grow other*** brassicas ***like*** cabbages, broccoli ***and*** brussels sprouts.

## *ROOTS*

Cabbage was probably domesticated from wild kale by the ancient Celts. The Romans selected and developed ever more varieties. Brussels sprouts were developed about 200 years ago in Belgium; broccoli was first produced about 150 years ago in an Italian market garden. It was a deep purple at first then the green we know today. Cauliflower is much older – beloved like cabbage in ancient Rome but originally domesticated – again from kale – in ancient Syria. The name cauliflower comes from cole – or kale – flower, as it's the early flower curd that's eaten.

## *MEDICINAL CABBAGES*

A warm cabbage leaf used to be applied to the breasts of women with mastitis, to ease the pain and inflammation. Certainly the warmth would help, but it is possible that cabbages also help heal skin problems – cabbage leaves and fresh cabbage juice have long been applied to wounds and skin irritations, and cabbage juice is mildly antiviral and antibacterial. A warm cabbage poultice is also said to ease the pain of arthritic joints.

Cabbages were also eaten to dispel drunkenness. While many other old remedies using cabbages – like drinking cabbage juice to expel worms – probably did work to varying degrees, this remedy probably didn't.

Cabbages were also used in ancient Rome to cure tumours and cancers – and do contain various anticancer and antioxidant compounds. It speeds up oestrogen metabolism, and helps inhibit breast cancer and pre cancerous polyp growth. In one study two tablespoons of cooked cabbage a day almost doubled the chances of avoiding stomach cancer.

Cabbage juice is mildly antibacterial and antiviral; eating cabbage has been shown to be helpful in diets of ulcer patients. Raw cabbage is probably better than cooked cabbage, (try fresh cabbage juice – but for medicinal rather than gourmet reasons) but cooked cabbage is also invaluable.

Eat lots.

Broccoli, brussels sprouts, chinese cabbage and caulies also share these properties to smaller or larger degrees. Broccoli is said to help lower blood pressure.

## *BRASSICA VARIETIES*

### *Chinese cabbage*

This can be grown at any time of the year; it matures very quickly. It makes a leafy but quite good coleslaw.

### *Red cabbage (e.g., Red Acre)*

These are usually large and are best planted in mid summer to mature in winter and spring. They make excellent coleslaw.

### *Savoy (e.g., Carter's improved)*

This is the crinkly cabbage. It is leafier and tenderer than most cabbages – and also less 'cabbagey' in flavour, so it is a much more seductive vegetable than ordinary cabbage.

### *Drumhead*

These are the big, solid cabbages – the sort you'd feed to a draught horse. They need to be sliced very finely for coleslaw or other salads or they are too tough.

***Sugarloaf***

These small, conical cabbages are 'one meal' cabbages. They also need to be sliced very finely and can be tough, though they are generally sweeter than the large drumheads.

***Broccoli***

*Italian calabrese* Pale green shoots with very tender side shoots. One of the most delicious broccolis.

*Romanesco* Spiralled heads – very attractive.

Also look for heat resistant hybrids.

***Cauliflower***

*Mini cauliflower* Excellent for growing in pots.

*Early purple head* Rich purple heads turn bright green when cooked.

*Paleleaf or paleface* An old-fashioned, slow maturing, very reliable cauliflower – our favourite.

*Snowball* Very fast-maturing caulie, but not suitable for hot districts.

## *CULTIVATION*

***Why you should grow your own***

Cauliflowers, etc. may be treated with a range of pesticides for cabbage aphids and caterpillars. Demeton-s-methyl is an organophosphate, extremely toxic to humans and birds (that eat the aphids and so are poisoned). It persists for several weeks. Dimenthoate is a suspected carcinogen; acephate is systemic, a new insecticide apparently with low persistence; permethrin is an artificial pyrethroid, relatively harmless except to bees and fish but quite persistent.

***Saving seed***

Cabbage, brussels sprouts, broccoli and caulies must be separated from each other – and other brassicas – and other varieties or they will cross. Collect seed only from non-hybrid plants. Pick out the top flowers and collect seed from the lower ones. Brussels sprouts and broccoli need to 'cross' with at least one other plant, preferably several, flowering at the same time.

Seeds last 3 to 4 years.

### *Sowing*

*Tropical areas*

*Cabbage* February to November.

*Broccoli* May to June.

*Brussels sprouts* Not suitable as they become puffy.

*Cauliflower* February to April.

*Subtropical areas*

*Cabbage* All year – choose varieties carefully for hot weather.

*Broccoli* All year – choose varieties carefully for hot weather.

*Brussels sprouts* Not suitable as they become puffy.

*Cauliflower* January to April.

*Temperate areas*

*Cabbage* July to March.

*Broccoli* Late December to May.

*Brussels sprouts* Late December to March.

*Cauliflower* Late December to March.

*Cool areas*

*Cabbage* August to March.

*Broccoli* October to February.

*Brussels sprouts* September to February.

*Cauliflower* September to January.

### *Germination and yield*

*Time taken to germinate*

This is between 4-24°C but it is best to sow when the temperature is over 16°C. Seeds emerge in 6 days.

*Time until first picking*

*Cabbage* 8 to 16 weeks.

*Broccoli* 12 to 16 weeks.

*Brussels sprouts* 16 to 20 weeks.

*Cauliflower* 14 to 26 weeks.

*Number of plants for a family of four*

This is difficult. You may eat 100 caulies a year – but if they all crop in a one month period you may only eat a small fraction of your crop. Try staggering your caulies, sowing no more than a dozen at once. In cool areas if your cauliflowers are going to mature in cool to cold weather, they'll keep for months – so you can plant as many as you think you'll eat in winter and spring.

Broccoli is easier. About a dozen plants, well fed, will feed a family of four – or two dozen if, like us, you like broccoli. Plant more every few months if the climate allows, so you get new luscious heads as well as the smaller regrowth.

About half a dozen brussels sprouts plants should be enough. (But I am biased – I don't really like brussels sprouts except stir-fried with almonds and olive oil). I like to have a cauli maturing every week – so that is fifty-two per year, but you will have to stagger the plantings carefully.

***Essential information***

Cabbages are an annual. Broccoli, caulies and brussels sprouts are biennial though they can become short-lived perennials if you stop them going to seed.

Grow the best variety for your climate and time of year. Protect from caterpillars. Feed well.

There is an enormous feeling of security in the sight of a garden filled with cabbages. They are perhaps the most domestic vegetable, giving a feeling of comfortable solidity. In fact I'm not all that keen on cabbages – or any of the brassicas – it's just I wouldn't feel right if I didn't grow them and eat one of them at least every two days with dinner. This affection for the cabbage family is probably something ingrained – part of the genes from innumerable cabbage eating ancestors.

The cabbage family has been one of the vegetable basics for centuries. It was loved by the ancient Romans and worshipped by the ancient Egyptians. Given cabbage's medical properties they may have had good reason.

***Growing***

Like most cottage staples cabbages should be incredibly hardy, and extraordinarily prolific. In Australia, however, cabbage growing has two drawbacks – it's often too hot to grow good ones (even 'cool weather' may have unseasonably hot days) – and our long seasons mean hatching after hatching of cabbage eating caterpillars.

The three rules for good cabbages (or broccoli, cauliflower, etc.) are:

- Plant them to mature in cool weather for the best tasting, firmest vegies – either late summer, autumn, winter or early spring
- Feed them well. Brassicas 'sulk' if they're not fed properly. I've had starved cabbages in a patch of the garden do nothing for two years – then suddenly decide to heart when I hadn't even bothered to look at them for months. You can in fact make use of this sulking habit – plant four seedlings together – the 'dominant' seedling will mature – but the others will wait till they have room and inclination – this is an easy way to stagger your crop with one planting
- Never plant a clump – or even worse – a row of cabbages. Don't plant them on the outskirts of the garden either. If you grow too many brassicas together it becomes a feast for the pests. Break them up with other plants.

### *Planting*

See above – but remember that even if you get a crop in hot weather, it won't taste as good as one harvested in the cool of the year. *Make sure you choose the right variety for your area and time of year.*

Timing is everything with brassicas. Look carefully at when they will mature so you don't get a glut of them. I try to time my brassicas to mature in early autumn, so we eat them all through winter and spring – then we forget about them for the rest of the year, except for the odd caulie and broccoli head and cabbage for coleslaw or stuffed cabbage. Actually, come to think of it, we eat quite a lot of brassicas all year round – but we really gorge on them in winter.

One way to stagger your plants is to plant more when they are about as tall as your hand. Another way is to plant different varieties with different maturing times so you get a long cropping period from one planting.

### *Feeding*

If you don't feed your brassicas they sulk – and you get a poor crop, or none at all.

Brassicas need lime, dolomite or wood ash in acid soil; they don't mature well in very acid soil or where the soil is deficient in calcium.

As most brassicas are slow growers they do well with a rich mulch that will provide nutrients all through their growing cycle, with a scatter of hen manure, blood and bone or soluble fertiliser when the plants are small if the soil is poor. An old-fashioned method of growing brassicas was to fill a trench with half sand and half rotted compost or manure and plant the brassicas on top.

Brassicas may fail to produce heads if the soil is deficient in calcium; they may turn slightly purple if they lack phosphorus; won't thrive with a lack of magnesium; and thin or twisted yellowed leaves and general poor growth and lack of hearting is usually due to molybdenum deficiency and is most common in caulies but can occur with brussels sprouts and to a lesser extent with all other brassicas. One ounce of molybdenum dissolved in hot water used as a foliar spray for every ten square yards of seedlings is effective. I use a green manure comfrey spray every day for a fortnight for a green foliar spray as long as I'm sure the leaves (ie the ones that have gone into the spray) aren't from a molybdenum scarce area. Leaves from old healthy caulies from the supermarket are a good source of a molybdenum rich material to use for a green foliar spray, or buy the trace element from your garden centre.

Remember with broccoli that the more you pick the heads the more you will have to feed the plant. I have harvested one broccoli plant for more than three years, picking the tiny heads every day – they toughen if you leave them any longer and let them flower. I fed the plant the best mulch I had – old lucerne that had been trodden and manured by chooks – and it kept producing wonderfully till we went on holidays and it went to seed. Old manure makes a good broccoli mulch. As an alternative a scatter of hen manure or blood and bone every fortnight.

An old way to grow brussels sprouts was to fill a trench with comfrey leaves, top with soil, leave for three weeks then plant the brussels sprout seedlings in the now sunken trench. Gradually fill the trench with a mulch of compost or old animal manure or more wilted comfrey leaves. This is a lot of work but you do get a wonderful crop of brussels sprouts, possibly because the roots are well aerated as well as fed. Otherwise give a light dressing of nitrogen rich fertiliser like hen manure, blood and bone or any of the quick fixes every two weeks till sprouts begin to form. Then stop.

Brussels sprouts are shallow rooted and a thick mulch is a good way to avoid moisture stress.

Cabbages like limed soil, but dolomite is better than lime as it can correct any tendency to magnesium deficiency. Wood ash will also make soil more alkaline and help relieve potash deficiency. Cabbages can be sown into a compost filled trench or a mulch of old animal manure suits them perfectly. In the absence of manure use the best mulch you have, with a dose of liquid manure or blood and bone, hen manure, etc. once a week. Early maturing varieties seem to need more fertilising than slower maturers, possibly because they don't have their large root systems. Cabbages need to be watered regularly, especially if they aren't mulched; alternating wet and dry will cause their heads to crack.

### *COMPANION PLANTING FOR CAULIES AND OTHER BRASSICAS*

The above may all sound complicated. In reality, if you have good soil and good cultivation practice, the only trick with brassicas is to know when to plant them and what varieties suit your area and the time of year you want to plant. That's mostly a matter of peering over your neighbour's shoulders and seeing what works for them – and looking through seed catalogues for appropriate varieties, rather than choosing the mass produced seedlings so often sold by nurseries, that are almost suitable for most areas – but really suitable for none.

The main reason for using companion planting with your brassicas is to disguise them so aphids and caterpillar producing butterflies won't find them.

Cabbage grown with red or white clover between the rows has fewer aphids and fewer cabbage white butterflies, partly due to camouflage but also partly due to an increase in pest eating predators, especially ground dwelling beetles and wasps. Try mowing your patch of clover very short, planting the seedlings in a long narrow trench (this is an exception to not planting in rows), then mulching them well to suppress the clover immediately around each seedling. Mow just either side of the trench – but let the rest flower.

The bacteria associated with the clover roots will also add nitrogen to the soil as the mown clover decomposes.

Lots of flowering weeds around the vegie garden will cut down the number of aphids on brassicas, by attracting predators who love the flowers, and who may also prefer to lay their eggs on the weeds.

Try a trap crop of brassicas gone to flower: aphids seem to prefer these plants and cabbage white butterflies may feed on the flowers then lay their eggs on the leaves – and leave your seedlings alone.

The scents of cabbages and tomatoes grown together help mask each other, and will reduce the number of aphids and, to a much lesser extent, cabbage white or cabbage moth caterpillars.

Other ways of discouraging butterflies include interplanting crops that disguise the smell or shape of the brassicas – the more plants the more disguise – and the fewer caterpillars. It's an almost direct correlation. Ten disguise plants to one cabbage will give you only a tenth of the caterpillars – more or less (hopefully less) depending on the disguise value of the other plants and the variety of the cabbages, the time of year and many other variables, including what weeds and other crops are grown nearby.

If nematodes are a problem try growing mustard in between the rows or grow mustard before the brassicas and slash it for mulch. Keep up levels of organic matter in the soil to encourage earthworms, mycelium webs and other ways of destroying young nematodes. Grow comfrey nearby for free good quality mulch.

### *Cabbages, caulies, etc. as herbicides*

Brassicas going too seed inhibit the germination of seeds around them and the growth of other plants. I make use of this by letting a plot of brassicas go to seed in spring – then hauling them out two months later. The result is a nearly weed free bed for early summer planting – and the massive roots have 'dug' the soil.

## *GROWING PAINS*

Pests find their food supply in two ways – either by scent or appearance – often by silhouette. Brassicas have a very distinctive shape. The more you interplant your cabbages, the less of a pest problem there'll be.

This year, for example, I've got one lot of broccoli planted on the terrace by the kitchen. It's an almost complete failure – the shapes are very visible to any pest that flutters by. And I have another lot disguised among parsnips and dahlias. They're doing fine – even though they are only a few metres away.

If you are really worried by caterpillars, ***make sure you let a few brassicas go to flower***.

Most pests are lazy – they'll lay their eggs where they feed. If you let a few broccoli plants flower – they'll last for years if you keep snipping them – you'll find most of the eggs are laid on them, after the butterflies have fed on the nectar from the flowers.

Our best defence here are the annual wild turnip weeds. They flower through most of summer, and their presence is enough to protect the cabbage crop nearby.

### ***Spindly broccoli***

This has been starved. Feed the poor thing and it'll feed you. (Old hen manure, etc. is excellent – broccoli need more nitrogen than other brassicas, as they give more crop per plant if you keep harvesting the heads.)

Don't just pick the central broccoli head. The more you pick your broccoli the more you'll get. The heads will be progressively smaller, but there'll be more and more of them. I once kept a broccoli plant going for three years. Then I went on holiday and the whole lot went to seed, and toughened. By then it was enormous. At the moment we've got rather dwarf looking cabbages that we've been harvesting for two and a half years. They produce small, brussels sprout like heads at irregular intervals.

### *Puffy brussels sprouts*

If your brussels sprouts aren't firm it's either too hot or you used too much nitrogen to feed them (mulch instead for both problems). In a trial plot here, compost fed sprouts planted at the same time as urea fed sprouts yielded an excellent crop – the urea fed crop gave a few puffy blobs then went to seed.

### *Puffy or gone-to-seed cabbage*

Cabbage can be sown at any warm time of the year, though the firmest heads come from cabbage planted after Christmas for autumn winter and spring. Cabbage can go to seed quickly in hot weather. Pick cabbages as soon as the head seems to elongate – at this stage it's getting ready to burst to seed. Puffy cabbage have had too much nitrogen and too much heat and water. Give a more balanced feed, especially if you like summer cabbage.

Like brussels sprouts, compost fed cabbage tolerates extremes more than cabbage fed on a high nitrogen fertiliser. If you must use a high nitrogen fertiliser like Dynamic Lifter or hen manure, try to give a fortnightly dose of liquid foliar seaweed spray to help check nutritional imbalances.

### *Purple or tough cauliflower*

Summer caulies turn purple and become tough. Wrap the outer leaves around them to keep them soft, white and tender (sounds like a detergent commercial for your hands). New varieties don't have enough leaves to wrap round the heart – avoid them. Beware of 'miracle maturers', too – caulies that are supposed to heart early. Most I've tried here have matured at the same rate as the non-hybrids – but only with enormous quantities of fertiliser and water. They don't hold as well as old-fashioned 'Paleface' either.

Try cutting off the head of the cauliflower – don't pull the whole thing up. Small heads should then form around the stalk. These can be eaten too. Once the stalk starts to rot, though, remove it – it will inhibit other plants.

### *Aphids*

Plant the caulies, cabbages etc later – you have probably planted them too early. Add potash to the soil with wood ash, comfrey or compost. Hose them strongly or make a spray of glue and water to suffocate them.

### *Molybdenum deficiency*

This mostly affects cauliflowers but other brassicas can also suffer. Plants are stunted and yellow, with thin or distorted leaves and may not produce worthwhile sprouts or centres.

Most Australian soils are at least slightly molybdenum deficient. Compost made from molybdenum deficient material will also be deficient.

The traditional cure is molybdate dissolved in hot water used as a foliar spray. Make a molybdenum spray by soaking comfrey or cauliflower leaves from the greengrocer in water till it turns pale green. Spray morning and dusk for three days then weekly.

### *Magnesium deficiency*

Cabbages are susceptible to magnesium deficiency. The most obvious symptom is brittle areas between the veins.

Give each plant a teaspoon full of dolomite, well watered in. Try foliar sprays if the plants are large.

### *Phosphorus deficiency*

Cabbages are pale and don't last.

Add ground rock phosphate or old hen manure.

### *Potash deficiency*

Brittle areas round the leaves.

Sprinkle wood ash and water well. Try a foliar spray for a short term solution.

### *Black cabbage rot*

Leaves develop V-shaped brown patches that become thin and brittle. Affected seedlings often die.

Practice crop rotation making sure that you clear all infected material from old crops. Cover ground with clear plastic for three weeks after an infection. Most good compost will inhibit black cabbage rot, especially if made with lucerne hay. A double strength garlic spray or chive spray may help.

***Cabbage white butterfly, cabbage moth caterpillars***
Skeletonised foliage; young plants may be eaten to the ground.

Surround the beds with strongly perfumed herbs like lavender, or interplant with almost any other crop – the more interplanting the smaller your problem will be. The moths and butterflies recognise their food supply by the scent and silhouette – if you can disguise the cabbages, etc. you'll protect your crop.

It is also a good idea to always leave some brassicas from last season going to seed – or plant some specially for that purpose six months before. The adults feed on the brassica blossom – then lay their eggs on the leaves below, ignoring your seedlings. Wild brassica weeds are also good 'trap crops' – I once grew commercial crops with no other protection than gone to seed brassicas and turnip weed nearby.

Once the caterpillars are attacking the plants, try squashing them. This seems laborious, but is actually much faster than you'd think. The squashed – stationary – caterpillars attract birds, wasps and other predators to feed on them – and they will start eating the live ones too. Encourage a good weed or bush community around your garden so you always have plenty of caterpillars around – and the predators to eat them. This will eliminate the lag between pest and predator build up.

Empty egg shells in the beds may sometimes outfox the butterflies as to their population density. Strips or beds of white clover around or between the crop may also deter them.

Try a tansy repellent – just cover tansy with boiling water, cool, strain and spray. As a final resort, spray with DIPEL or derris. Make sure that you spray or dust the undersides of leaves as well as tops, as this is where the young caterpillars will be hiding.

Try flour first. This is a caterpillar stomach poison. It will take three or four days to be effective, however, and may be washed off before enough is eaten.

Mix flour and boiling water to a bill sticker's paste, then add more water and spay that. Glued up bugs stop eating – and are easy for predators to find.

Try DIPEL as the next resort, or clay spray (this is just clay and water – no dirt, though), bug juice or white pepper spray. (White pepper spray will slightly dehydrate the caterpillars. Most will die; the rest will be easy prey for birds, etc.).

You might also try dusting the leaves with powdered rock phosphate for the same effect. If these fail try wormwood spray, garlic, quassia, or dusting or spraying with derris. These are all last resorts, though, as they all kill non target species.

*Caterpillar trap*

This may be useful for large infestations where caterpillars denude one plant then move on to the next. Place a small three sided box at the base of plants – about 10 mm high. Place a scatter or lime or wood ash inside. The caterpillars should shelter there during the day and dehydrate. A scatter of wood ash around plants also stops migration.

*Note*: While the cabbage moth is quite different from the cabbage white butterfly – it's greyish brown and hairy with yellow diamond shaped markings when the wings are folded – the caterpillars of both are easily confused. Both are green and both devastate cabbages, cauliflowers and similar crops. Cabbage moth caterpillars however are a clearer green than cabbage white caterpillars and lack the velvety appearance and yellow stripe.

In terms of garden control however the difference is slight. Cabbage moths also lay their eggs on the underside of leaves. The cabbage moth caterpillar tends to eat towards the heart of the vegetable and may cause even more damage than the cabbage white.

Like cabbage whites, the cabbage moth caterpillars are predated by a range of imported wasps – different ones from the cabbage white's. Native wasps don't appear to be so particular and I have noticed two species here that will carry off either. The same range of birds also appears to attack both.

***Yellow or purple cauliflower heads***

These have been exposed to too much direct sunlight. Curl the leaves over while they are maturing.

### *Loose broccoli heads*

Pick them sooner, grow in cooler weather or choose a heat resistant variety.

### *Clubroot*

Roots are large and knobby; plants may wilt, especially in hot weather, die or just grow slowly.

Protect your crop from nematodes with a companion crop of crotalaria or mustard. Keep up levels of organic matter, especially in sandy areas where clubroot is worst. *You must always have organic matter steadily decomposing on top of the soil to control clubroot.*

Try barriers of old tin cans with tops and bottoms cut out as 'root guards'. Add a sprinkle of lime or dolomite to the soil to reduce acidity. Practice stringent crop rotation – at least four years before any of the cabbage family, swedes or turnips are grown in that spot.

### *Slugs*

Slugs love cabbages. Put a sharp collar made from an old tin can lid around each cabbage stalk or even a ring of much crinkled alfoil. Drizzle derris spray through the leaves, so it penetrates as much as possible – but wash very well before using as the derris may not break down as quickly in the shelter of the cabbage leaves. See 'Snails and slugs'.

## *FROM THE GARDEN TO THE TABLE*

### *The harvest*

Pick cabbages while they are still firm, they'll stay firm for months in cold or cool weather, but may quickly go to seed in hot weather. Some varieties 'hold' better than others. Pick cabbage as soon as it's firm in wet or humid weather, in case it starts to rot.

Once you've picked the first cabbage head baby ones sometimes appear on the stalk. These are also good to eat. Try them stir fried.

Pick broccoli as soon as the heads are big enough to bother with. Don't leave them too long as the texture coarsens and they open further to finally turn into yellow flowers. By this time they are tough, soggy and slightly 'off' tasting.

Don't just pick the first main great big head of broccoli. Once you've picked that one more will form at the sides – and once you've picked those you'll get still more – for years if you keep picking.

In hot weather you *must* pick broccoli every day – or every second day at most – or it will toughen. In cool weather a head may last for a couple of weeks without picking.

Caulies are best small too – they are firmest and sweetest then. Don't get greedy and wait for them to get bigger and bigger – you probably won't eat the whole thing anyway. Eat it when it's small and firmest and very white and the flowers are still curled into each other.

Pick brussels sprouts as soon as they're walnut size. They can soon get puffy and the leaves will be flabby and rank. The bottom ones are often too puffy to bother with.

Old-fashioned brussels sprout varieties crop over at least a month with the lower ones ready first, but modern varieties – bred for farmers who want to pick the whole lot and sell them and get the ground ready for another crop – often mature almost all at once.

*Fresh eating period* All year round.

*Storage Time* Several weeks in fridge. Store cabbages and broccoli and caulies in crumpled up newspaper – it will keep them dry and stop them smelling – and if they do smell it will stop the stink contaminating anything else.

*Nutritional value*

*Cabbage* 100 kj per 100 g good vitamin C, reasonable calcium and fibre.

*Broccoli* 150 kj per 100 g, excellent source of folic acid, vitamin A and C, good source of calcium and fibre.

*Brussels sprouts* 200 kj per 100 g, excellent vitamin C, folic acid and fibre.

*Caulies* 100 kj per 100 g, good vitamin C, reasonable folic acid and fibre.

*What parts you can eat*

All parts of brassicas are edible – except perhaps the roots. (These aren't toxic but aren't appetising either). Eat the heads – cabbage, caulie, etc. You can also eat the stalks – peel away the tough outside and stir fry the tender inside. You can also do this to the stalk as it goes to seed.

The flowers are good stir fried.

*Note*: If you don't like the 'cooked cabbage' – or broccoli, brussels sprouts, etc. smell – add a whole unshelled walnut to the water you boil it in – or of course stir fry instead.

*SAUERKRAUT*

This can also be made with lettuce or cabbage or young green beans.

Shred clean crisp cabbage as finely as you can. Weigh out two kilos in a bowl and cover with three tablespoons of salt. Mix and leave till the cabbage wilts a bit – it is easier to press into a jar when soft and the juice should start flowing. Now press down as hard as you can in a pottery or opaque plastic jar. Try to force all air out – this will also help to force the juice out. Cover with a plastic bag half filled with water – this should edge snugly round the cabbage so no air can get in at all. If there isn't enough juice to cover the cabbage in 24 hours add salt and water – one cup of salt to ten cups of water. Leave in a cool place (no more than 25°C) for about six weeks. Then place in a saucepan with the juice and bring to the boil. Pack into clean jars and seal.

*How to cook sauerkraut.*

Melt a knob of butter in a large pan; sauté a sliced onion till transparent. Rinse and drain the sauerkraut and cook for five minutes, add a grated apple. Simmer for 30 minutes. A little stock or water will be needed to moisten. Bake in a moderate oven till tender.

Sauerkraut can be sprinkled with brown sugar or caraway seeds.

*RED CABBAGE SALAD*

This is simply made as follows: Dress your finely chopped red cabbage with a very little sesame oil and soy sauce (a teaspoon of each is plenty for three cups of cabbage); then dust with toasted sesame seeds.

*PICKLED CABBAGE*

Slice, sprinkle with salt, stand for twelve hours, press out moisture, place in jars and cover with vinegar. Seal the jars.

*DRIED CABBAGE*

This is usually made from Chinese cabbage, though other cabbages can be used as well – choose tender inner leaves for drying. You can brush the leaves with lemon juice first – it keeps its colour and softness better – but isn't necessary. Leave the leaves in the sun for a couple of days till they are almost transparent. Take them in at night.

Brush the dried leaves with water and fill with vinegar rice with a layer of pickles in the middle. Wrap in a neat package and slice thinly, so you see a green then a white then a pickle layer.

*VINEGAR RICE*

For every two cups of rice add two tablespoons of white vinegar and half a tablespoon of sugar.

*RUMBLEDETHUMPS*

2 cups mashed potato
2 cups cooked cabbage
1 chopped onion, sautéed in butter
grated sharp cheese
pepper

Mix all the ingredients except the cheese. Place in the oven, top with cheese. Bake till hot.

*COLESLAW*

This is basically cabbage shredded as finely as possible, dressed either with – usually bottled – mayonnaise or vinaigrette dressing. I prefer the latter. You can use any of the cabbages for coleslaw, including red cabbage and Chinese cabbage.

Try adding:

- grated carrot and/or grated beetroot
- chopped parsley
- a little chopped dill
- sesame seeds

- walnuts and thinly sliced unpeeled apple
- roughly chopped macadamias
- thinly sliced smoked pork with thinly sliced granny smith apple
- raisins (a popular addition, though I don't like them)

*CABBAGE WITH ONIONS AND OPTIONAL BACON*

Fry a few onions in oil; add a little chopped bacon, then add finely shredded cabbage. Stir till cooked, then add just a dash of soy sauce.

Some chilli and garlic added with the bacon is a good addition too.

*STIR FRIED BRUSSELS SPROUTS WITH ALMONDS.*

Brussels sprouts get even soggier on contact with water. (*Note*: cold climate brussels sprouts are firmer – we don't get very good ones here. If I lived in Tasmania I might love brussels sprouts more.)

Heat olive oil in a pan, add chopped garlic, then throw in brussel spouts – not too many or they will steam instead of fry. Cook, stirring rapidly, till they turn bright green, then another five minutes. Add peeled sliced or whole almonds and cook another minute. Serve hot.

This is also good with cauliflower.

*CAULIFLOWER SALAD*

Steam cauli florets till *just* tender. Cool under cold water at once. Dress with one part lemon juice, three parts olive oil and a good dash of grainy French mustard and a generous dash of garlic. Now add lots of chopped parsley and garlic chives – and serve either semi-warm or cold.

# *corn*

***If you can grow*** Corn ***you can grow*** Maize ***and*** Popcorn

### *CORN ROOTS*

In ancient North America a beautiful woman appeared to a young warrior, her hair was wild and gold. She beckoned to him and whispered to him to set the prairie on fire and drag her by the hair through the burnt grass.

The young man was apparently familiar with peculiar desires, because he obeyed her without question; and wherever he dragged her corn sprang up, with a tuft of the woman's hair in every cob to remind the man and his people of her gift to them.

This is just one of the legends of North and South America of the coming of corn – though the name corn was given to it by English settlers, who called it Indian corn – corn had previously referred to wheat. (In animal husbandry it meant oats . . . yes, I know this is confusing. It was then too.)

According to Captain John Smith (the one defended by Pocohontas): 'Their cone they roast in the eare greene and brusing it in a mortar with a Polt . . . and so boyle it for a dainte.'

Corn was probably first domesticated – or picked wild – in the south and spread through Mexico where it is still a staple, up through the Americas. Many South American cultures believed corn was a gift from the gods – or holy itself – or that humans raised themselves from animal to human by learning to grow maize. (Note that the Mexican word for maize is mays.)

Christopher Columbus brought corn (as well as tomatoes and potatoes and chilies) to Europe. It was accepted rapidly, but mostly used for stock food or ground into corn flour or used for cooked dishes like polenta by Europeans until the Amerindians taught them the joys of corn on the cob. The word corn comes from 'carnus' meaning meat; in other words, corn is poor man's meat, a staple food around a large part of the world. In fact it became so popular as a cheap and filling way to feed poor folk that Europe experienced an epidemic of pellagra shortly after its introduction due to nutritional deficiencies.

## *CORN AND HEALTH*

Eating a corn rich diet has been linked with a lower rate of cancer, and a greater resistance to various virus diseases, possibly due to corn's protease inhibitors. Corn is one of the staples of people with coeliac disease – a gluten intolerance. Like all the major foods, however, a small proportion of the population may be intolerant of it: in susceptible people only it can precipitate attacks of rheumatoid arthritis or migraines. Large amounts should be avoided by diabetics.

### *Corn for cystitis*

If you are troubled by cystitis – burning urine – save your corn tassels, and either use them fresh or dry them for winter use. Make a tea by covering one cup of tassels with one cup boiling water. Leave till cool, then drink a cup every hour. It will soothe the inflamed tissues – definitely not a cure for cystitis but a welcome relief. (See your doctor – cystitis can lead to kidney failure – and if you get it repeatedly change doctors until you get one that will investigate *why* you keep getting it.)

If you have had recurrent cystitis and are sensitive to acid drinks like fruit juice, regularly drinking corn silk tea will help soothe – but avoid the acid too for a while.

## *SOME CORN VARIETIES*

### *Hybrid*

*Rosella* Once a variety grown mostly for processing, this is a very reliable corn with even cobs.

*Miracle* Matures in 65 to 80 days, and will crop even under poor conditions.

*Honeysweet improved* This has a very high sugar content and stays sweet for a week after harvest.
*Snogold* Another very sweet variety with white and gold kernels, this is my favourite corn.

### *Open pollinated*

*Golden bantam* This will give you at least two, if not four cobs per stalk – a reasonably early and prolific cropper.
*Mexican sweet corn* This is a deep yellow red colour – lovely as long as you pick it young enough.
*Balinese corn* A majestic plant, up to three metres high, with two good cobs per plant – a good crop to boast about in the back garden.

### *Popcorns*

Most seed companies have a popcorn-like hybrid. Snowpop that will give you nice pale balls when you pop it. Eden Seeds and Phoenix (see page 163) have more interesting varieties – look for red or blue popping corn. (Who needs artificial colouring?)

### *Maize*

Maize gives bigger crops, longer stalks and larger cobs than sweet corn. If you are growing corn for chooks, grow maize for a larger harvest. Look for blue or red maize, or a silage corn like 'Golden Superb'.

### *Ornamental corn*

This is a form of maize. Each cob is different – red or multi-coloured with bits of blue, red or orange – great heaped in bowls on the table. You can eat ornamental corn as long as you pick it young enough – and the chooks love the mature cobs if some are too tatty to keep for decoration. A great gift too.

## *CULTIVATION*

### *Why you should grow your own*

Corn will probably have been treated for heliothis caterpillars with Endosulphan – an organochlorine with a half life of 2 to 4 weeks.

is extremely toxic to birds that may eat infected caterpillars as well as being directly affected through skin absorption. Endosulphan is also toxic to fish if it enters waterways from run off.

### *Essential information*

Corn is a grass – it's very hard to overfeed it. It does best with lots of water but can also be grown as a drought crop. Pick it young and sweet, eat it at once and plant some more.

Different varieties of corn are used for different purposes – thinned skin corn for grinding into cornflour, hard corn for cracking and using as stock food, small round hard kernels for coarsely grinding into polenta and cornmeal, 'popping' corn with small hard kernels with a high starch content and tiny air pockets in them, so they 'pop' when they're heated – and sweet corn, which is the corn we are most familiar with.

All the different corns or maizes are tender enough to gnaw on when young, but only sweet corn stays soft and sweet and milky when mature. (If you want to eat maize like sweet corn you need to pick it before any of the kernels turn fully yellow.)

Corn starts to lose its sweetness as soon as it is picked – which is why, if you've never run (not walked – run) with freshly picked corn to a pot of boiling water and dunked it in, then hauled it out two minutes later and eaten the lot with melted butter and black pepper – well, you haven't tasted corn.

Modern varieties of corn make up for the loss of sweetness by being extra sweet to begin with. But corn's texture changes too, as it gets older – and there are other flavours that get lost too, not just the sweetness. Fresh – very fresh – corn is one of the glories of the world – and if you don't grow your own you'll never know it.

Corn is also one of the 'boasting' plants in the vegie garden – tall and beautiful and easy for any passer-by to admire. It can be one of the loveliest of all vegetables, with its leafy spearheads and silky tassels, especially with colourful vegetables like bright stalked Swiss chard, red leafed lettuce or golden calendulas below it.

### *Corn seed*

Corn seed is easy to keep – you just have to leave it on the stalk till the 'paper' around it browns off and the corn inside is hard and deep yellow. I keep our seed corn on the cobs till I need it, then just rub it off next spring between my fingers.

However, most corn sold today is hybridised and won't come true to type, unless you have bought open pollinated seed from a seed merchant that specialises in old varieties. Even if you do have open pollinated corn, it may still cross with any other corn grown nearby – either your own or your neighbour's – so you have to keep it isolated. Corn is pollinated by the wind, so you need to grow your corn at least 500 metres from any other variety – or even one kilometre away in windy areas where there aren't any windbreaks of belts of trees or hills.

*You can also try the paper bag trick*

Corn produces pollen on the male tassel on top of the plant. You need to place paper bags over all the cobs you want to save seed from *before* the tassels emerge. Collect the pollen by shaking the bags slightly on a hot day.

Now blow the collected pollen – a soft golden dust – onto the female parts of the corn – the cob with the silken tassels. *Every* tassel must be pollinated with the pollen, or some of the kernels won't be filled.

Put the paper bag back over the corn so it doesn't get pollinated by something else.

Of course you can also play around with cross pollinating, and try deliberately crossing varieties – or just use your corn seed anyway. I did that several years in a row, saving seed from hybrid varieties as well as cross pollinated, open pollinated varieties. The result was a maize like corn the next year – one a sort of dull orange, one very long and thin, one pure white and incredibly tough – but never corn to salivate over, though the chooks loved it.

Sweet corn seed lasts two or three years, though you can be lucky and have it still germinate after a decade – just don't rely on it. Popcorn and hard corn varieties generally last much longer than sweet corn seed.

### *Sowing time*

*Tropical areas* All year round.
*Subtropical areas* June to February, after soils warm up.
*Temperate areas* September to January or February if you are prepared to cosset it – see below.
*Cool areas* October to December or January if it's hot and you are prepared to cosset it – see below.

### *Germination and yield*

*Temperatures* 20-35°C.
*Seedlings emerge* 6 to 14 days.
*Time to first picking* 12 to 16 weeks (depends on warmth and variety).
*Number of plants needed for a family of four* Each stalk will give from 1 to 3 cobs, depending on variety, warmth and feeding. Work out how many you want to eat.
*Successions* Plant at least three crops of corn or a patch every 2 to 3 weeks for avid corn eaters, or plant more when the first lot are almost to your knees.

### *Planting*

Sow seed in spring after frosts have finished (or once the soil has warmed up enough to sit on it comfortably) – and then protect the corn seedlings from late frosts with old plastic bottles with the bottoms cut out (like miniature greenhouses). These also keep away snails (and cut worms too if you press them into the soil). Then plant more every fortnight until early autumn, so you get a continuous supply.

In cool areas this means you can plant corn from about October/ November to December; in warmer areas September to January; and in subtropical to tropical areas August to February. (See below for growing corn slightly out of season.)

Corn seed is normally planted 5 to 8 cm deep, with 30 cm between the plants. Some desert Amerindians however planted it a foot deep – the sandy soil insulated it and its roots, so that it survived desert temperatures and long periods without rain.

Don't plant your corn in rows – remember, it is pollinated by the wind. Plant it close together in a block instead or you won't get well filled cobs.

Corn takes from 60 to 110 days to mature, depending on the variety and the weather. The more sun, the sweeter the corn – so early maturing varieties won't be as full of flavour as later maturing ones. They are also likely to be much smaller and only produce 1 to 2 cobs per stalk. Later maturing ones can produce 3 to 4, and even up to six.

### *Growing*

Think of corn as a grass. It is in fact a grass – its ancestor is teosinte, a tall grass with narrow corn-like ears. It needs plenty of feeding and lots of water to bear well. There is no point in trying to make your corn diet. You won't get any corn cobs.

Corn is a very heavy feeder. It is also shallow rooted, which means that it can be grown even on poor soil if you are prepared to feed it as it grows. To control weeds, mulch corn as soon as it is as thick as your little finger. This is essential – if you don't mulch you'll have to weed: corn won't stand any competition. If possible, keep it mulched up to leaf level for best results – but most people won't have this much mulch. Give it a sprinkle of fertiliser or home-made liquid manure – or even urine diluted with 10 parts water – every week until the tassels start to form. Then don't feed it any more.

Corn slightly inhibits the growth of many plants around it. I grow climbing beans up my corn. They don't crop as well, but do crop slightly sooner, and the bean nodules give back some of the nitrogen the hungry corn crop is taking.

Don't leave corn stalks to dry out when you have picked the corn. If you pick them when they're still quite green and soft they will break down faster as mulch or compost.

#### *Watering corn*

Corn does well with lots of water – and water is a scarce commodity. Use water ***under*** the mulch or use drip irrigation. However, high humidity also helps corn pollination – so when the tassels are forming use overhead watering instead.

### *Other ways to grow corn*

#### *Corn in weed mat*

Spread weed mat over a spare bit of sunny lawn. Weigh it down so it doesn't blow away. Cut egg-sized holes every 30 cm and scoop out the grass and soil with a spoon. Plant one seed or seedling per hole. Feed with liquid manure every week. The corn will grow slowly for the first few weeks till the grass breaks down – then it will gallop away.

You can take away the weed mat at the end of the growing season. You'll be left with a nice bare space to grow onions.

#### *Corn in tyres*

This is good for growing corn in winter (see below) or if you are afraid of late frosts.

Place one tyre on top of another. Place spadefuls of compost or potting mix inside all around the edge and in the middle – a bit like the spokes on a bicycle – then plant the seed or seedling. Keep moist. You'll get a clump of fast, tall-growing corn. Mulch it regularly as it grows till the tyres are full of mulch.

#### *Trenched corn*

This is a good method for growing corn through very hot, dry summers.

Dig a trench about a spade's depth and width. Line it with compost to about half way up the sides. Plant your corn seeds about 30 cm apart. Cover with just a little compost. Now fill in the trench with sand.

When the corn pokes its head up, mulch it very well with loose, dry material, right up to leaf height – old bracken or very old straw is excellent.

Grown this way corn will crop even where there is almost no rain the entire summer. I know – it was my main food source in the worst year of the last drought.

#### *Growing corn through frosty winters*

I have managed to grow corn here all year round, with the temperature descending to minus 5°C in winter. I don't know if it was worth the trouble – after all, corn for cooking and animals is easily stored. But the fresh cobs of corn were a treat in late winter and spring – even if they were fairly tasteless by home-grown corn-on-the-cob standards, they were still better than frozen corn.

Plant your main lot of corn in spring. I find the first lot matures unevenly, so your crop will be staggered over about a month. Plant the next lot about six weeks later, then plant at three weekly intervals. An alternative is to plant both early, mid-season and late-maturing varieties of corn at the same time, then more about Christmas.

If you want to 'overwinter' corn, plant more in late summer, about one month before the first frost. As soon as the soil starts to cool down, and trees begin to show their colours, mulch the corn heavily – very heavily – right up to the tips of the green leaves.

Mulch attracts frost and the leaves above it will tend to freeze. With this method there are no leaves above it – or almost none. Push the mulch down on sunny days, and fluff it right up at night. The trapped air will insulate the plants and the soil and stop both from freezing.

Another alternative is to throw old tyres over each corn plant – or plant your corn in the tyres to begin with, about two plants per tyre. Keep piling on the tyres as they grow – keep throwing in mulch as you put on the tyres. With this method you don't have to entirely cover the plant – the black will absorb warmth and the tyres will insulate – and make sure that the mulch is well below the level of the tyre. I find a quick-growing crop of radish, thrown around the corn on a bit of soil on top of the mulch, also reduces frost damage.

The corn will mature very slowly – and won't be very sweet. But for corn addicts, year round fresh corn is possible, even in frosty areas.

## *COMPANION PLANTING WITH CORN*

In three trials here I've found that corn is stunted by growing with or next to sunflowers.

In my garden corn seems to do best with beans. Corn planted

with beans seems to increase the number of predators for both plants. Corn grows well with cucumbers, but the cucumbers become prone to powdery mildew. Pumpkin grown with corn keeps down weeds – this was a traditional Mexican form of companion planting. The shapes of pumpkin and corn together appear to confuse pests and interfere with the budworm moth's flight path.

Cotton and sesame have been grown commercially with corn in the USA to control budworms by attracting more predators. Peanuts grown with corn increase the number of spiders – partly because they have more shelter – leading to fewer borers and other pests. Plant the peanuts at the same time as the corn, in early spring, and use the old corn stalks as mulch for the ripening peanuts.

## *GROWING PAINS*

### *Poor pollination*

This causes cobs to have gaps between the kernels – sometimes only a few kernels on the cob will be 'filled'.

Corn should be planted in blocks at least one metre wide to help pollination. The male tassel on top of the corn stalk produces pollen which must be shed onto the 'silk' below. If you have already planted your corn in one long row, you can place a brown paper bag over some of the male tassels; shake the tassel well inside the bag, then lightly shake the pollen onto the silks. Occasionally, male tassels finish producing their pollen before the silks are ready below. If this happens, try and find another crop of corn and 'borrow' some pollen.

High humidity will help pollination: overhead water in the morning onto mulch, so that the moisture evaporates all day. Growing corn close together will also raise humidity – as will growing tomatoes nearby.

### *Hard corn*

This is produced by maize, not sweet corn. Maize is only tender when very young. Occasionally sweet corn seed is mixed with maize seed, or has been collected from maize plants accidentally

– sometimes because their parent has been cross-pollinated by maize or some other genetic accident. Feed the hard corn to the hens or grind it for polenta or add it to long cooking stews. There is nothing you can do to make it softer on the plant. (People used to add ashes to the water when boiling maize to soften it, but this is not recommended nowadays.)

### *Caterpillars and corn ear worm*

Heliothis caterpillars burrow into the ears and eat the kernels. They can be difficult to get at and the tough covering of the ear protects them from predators, dusts and sprays. They tend to fly at dusk when predators aren't active. Spiders are the best budworm control – never destroy a spider's web near your garden.

Check ears for droppings and 'sawdust' like deposits. Remove the outer coverings, squash the pest, then smooth everything back into place. Injections of oil spray behind the covering may be effective but squashing is surer and less work. Alternatively, wipe the silk with mineral oil once a week to deter them. Try a tansy repellent spray (just cover tansy with boiling water; cool and strain) in the early morning so the silk has a chance to dry out by mid-morning. (If it stays wet and claggy you may get poor pollination.)

A high bird population and having flowering parsnips or other flowering umbelliferae around the crop to attract wasps, hoverflies, spiders and other predators is the best prevention. The more spiders you have the fewer caterpillars will eat your corn. We had enormous problems with heliothis caterpillars here until I began letting large numbers of parsnips flower.

See also under companion planting.

### *Eelworm, cutworm, nematodes*

These cause young plants to die, apparently cut at the bottom.

Compost is the best long-term cure – or any mulch that will rapidly decompose. Add a scatter of pelletised hen manure or other high-nitrogen material on top of the mulch to encourage it to break down quickly. Always keep up levels of organic matter, especially in sandy soil.

As a short term measure, stake each seedling with two toothpicks so it can't be cut, or place each seedling in its own miniature greenhouse made out of the top of an old plastic bottle. (This will also speed up growth.) Drizzle a molasses solution round the plants. Try a green manure mustard crop before sowing large crops of corn in sandy areas. It only takes six to eight weeks to grow mustard for green manure. Help it to break down with a scatter of hen manure or even sulphate of ammonia – may be not organic, but in this case effective.

## *FROM THE GARDEN TO THE TABLE*

Corn is one of the world's great staples – for making porridge, cornbread, polenta, adding to soups and stews and feeding to stock.

But the best way to eat corn is always fresh – bung it in boiling water, cook it for two minutes (or from five to ten minutes if it's older), then eat it hot with plenty of butter or margarine, or even garlic-impregnated olive oil, and a generous grating of black pepper. Don't add salt to the water when cooking corn – it makes the kernels tough. Add salt later if you are a salt addict.

### *The harvest*

*Fresh eating period* Frost free period minus 100 days.
*Storage time* Several weeks in fridge; can be frozen or dried. If you need to keep your corn, wrap it in a wet teatowel or newspaper and keep it in the fridge, still in its papery wrapping.
*Food value* 348 kj per 100 g (or much more if you count the butter you'll slather over it). Good source of vitamin A, potassium, calcium, phosphorus and a little protein.

#### *When to pick corn*

Corn is ready when the kernels are filled – but if you wait too long the corn gets tougher and starchier, and not as sweet. Check the tassels first – when they *just* start to dry off, peel back the papery covering and look at the top of the cob (squash any lingering caterpillars). When the kernels are yellowish just below the tip – but not quite at the tip – pick at once and race it to the pot.

Another way to check ripeness is to squeeze one of the kernels. If it's milky, the cob is ready to eat.

### *Corn dollies*

Note that corn dollies are also made from wheat stalks and heads – several grains are referred to as 'corn'.

Corn dollies were once part of a fertility rite – the last and strongest stalk of corn was saved to make an image of the goddess to watch over the harvest until the next year.

Cut the cob out of its paper, but leave the paper intact. Leave it to dry thoroughly.

Now turn it upside down, so the end of the stalk is on top. Take another piece of corn paper from another corn cob, twist it into a rope and tie it a few centimetres below the stalk. This is the 'head'. Now tie another strand half way down – and you have a waist.

From here on it's up to you. Trim the 'head'; paint on a face; twist out plaited legs and arms or paint a skirt or divide the base into trousered legs; glue on a wig made of plaited corn paper or even dried tassels.

Hang up your dollies over the door or on a shelf where they can see who comes in the front door, to protect your home from harm – and to ensure a fertile harvest next year.

### ***Using maize***

Maize kernels used to be softened for eating by adding an alkali to the water – either heated limestone or roasted snail shells (minus the snail) or very very fine grinding. I have used our coffee grinder to grind a very rough cornmeal.

### ***Dealing with a surplus***

Corn can be dried simply by leaving it on the stalk. In rainy weather bend the stalk over so the cobs point downwards and the water runs off them, instead of soaking into the top.

When you pick them don't bother to scrape off the kernels, unless you are short of storage space. Just keep the whole cob, paper wrapping and all – but make sure both the kernels inside and the wrapping are quite dry before you store them.

Use the dried kernels in soups and stews – they need about two hours soaking and about half an hour's cooking. Give surplus cobs to the hens (a free-ranging hen needs about a cob a day). Dry the kernels and grind them for cornflour later.

If you have a lot of fresh corn, 'milk' the kernels and freeze the juice – add to any soup or stew for protein and thickening.

*MICROWAVED CORN*

Cut the stalk off the corn so it fits in the microwave. Leave the papery leaves on. Stick it on high for ten minutes – then unwrap and eat.

*BARBECUED CORN*

Soak the corn cobs, papery wrapping and all, for ten minutes, then cook on a hot barbecue for about ten minutes each side. Unwrap and eat hot.

*CORN AND EGG SOUP*

Scrape the kernels off three raw cobs of corn into three cups of chicken stock. Simmer for five minutes. Add one teaspoon chopped parsley or fresh coriander, one teaspoon chopped chives. Beat an egg in a cup, add one teaspoon of arrowroot and mix well, then pour it into the hot stock, stirring madly all the time. Take off the heat at once, and serve hot, with lots of black pepper. The fresher the corn, and the better the stock, the better this soup is.

*CREAMED CORN*

Forget about that horrible stuff in cans. Melt one dessertspoon of butter in a saucepan. Add one dessertspoon of plain flour, and mix well. Stir in a cup of cream, mix until smooth, then mix in the kernels scraped off six cobs of corn.

Heat gently, stirring till thick, for about five minutes. Add more cream if it thickens too much. Take off the heat. Add a small squeeze of lemon juice, lots of black pepper – and eat hot. Forget about the soggy toast – it doesn't need it.

*CORN AND BEANS*

Corn and red kidney beans together are said to make a 'complete' protein, essential for vegetarians. They also taste good together.

Sauté two chopped onions and twenty cloves of garlic (no, this isn't a misprint – don't worry you'll hardly taste it) in a quarter of a cup of olive oil. When soft, add two cups of kidney beans – either canned or soaked overnight and simmered till tender – plus either six tomatoes peeled and chopped, or a can of tomatoes. Simmer twenty minutes, add the kernels scraped off four cobs of corn. Simmer another fifteen minutes; add more tomato if the mixture gets too thick. Add black pepper or chilli to taste at the end of cooking. (If you really love chilli throw in a couple when you sauté the garlic.)

Serve hot.

*POPCORN*

Pick the corn when its well filled and firm and let it dry quite hard before you use it. Then heat a pan (with lid) smear the bottom with oil or butter, bung in your popcorn – not too much or it won't heat evenly – and remember that it swells a lot on cooking. Shake like mad till the lot has popped. Add salt and more butter if you're greedy – or toss it in a little uncooled toffee mixture for corn candy.

Popcorn is actually good for you as long as you don't overdo the butter and salt – use canola margarine instead and a bit of black pepper instead of salt, or a dust of chilli if you like your food fiery. Avoid movie popcorn though – it's made with saturated fat and filled with enough cholestrol and calories to sink the Lusitania. (It's said that most of Elvis Presley's bulk was popcorn – or the fat that he ate with it. If Elvis had had a teflon frypan, who knows, history may have been different.)

*CORN MEAL AND CHERRY CAKE*

This is delicious – light and fruity.

1 cup (200 g) corn meal
1½ cups milk
½ cup fresh orange juice
1 cup brown sugar

½ cup caster sugar
2 eggs
1½ cups self-raising flour
grated zest of three oranges
1 cup crystallised cherries, finely chopped

Place the milk, cornmeal, orange juice, caster sugar and orange zest in a saucepan. Simmer for five minutes. Stir all the time so it doesn't stick. Take off the heat and leave till cool.

Beat butter and brown sugar till smooth. Add the eggs one at a time and beat till smooth again. Fold in the flour then the cornmeal mixture and the chopped cherries.

Bake in a moderate oven for one and a quarter hours or till a skewer comes out clean. Leave in the pan for ten minutes. Sift icing sugar over it while it is still warm, or wait till it is cool and ice with a very little almond icing at the edges.

*PARCHED CORN*

Leave some cobs on the stalk till they are dry, cut off with a knife, then leave in a sealed container in the fridge – they should keep for three months or more. Fry them in oil like popcorn. They won't pop properly – they'll be more chewy, but I prefer them like that. A bit of garlic added to the oil is good, as is a touch of pepper afterwards.

*CORNMEAL*

This is usually made from maize but will also work with sweet corn. Let the kernels dry on the cob till hard. Scrape them off and store in jars or a dry place till needed. You can use a grain mill to grind them or even a kitchen blender or a coffee grinder.

*CORNMEAL MUSH*

For each person, put into a saucepan three quarters of a cup of boiling water and a quarter of a cup of corn meal. Boil for three minutes, stirring well. Add more water if you want a thinner mush. Eat the mush hot with honey and cream, or add melted butter and black pepper, or serve with tomato sauce. Cornmeal mush can also be left to cool, then sliced thinly and fried in butter – lovely.

*CORNMEAL BREAD*

1 cup coarse corn meal
one and a half cups plain flour
3 teaspoons baking powder
1 egg
1 cup milk
2 tablespoons melted butter

Mix the butter, egg and milk. Fold in the dry ingredients. Bake in a hot oven for 25 minutes. It is ready when the top springs back when pressed.

Eat hot, eat cold, wonderful with cheese or just butter. Freezes well.

*RICH BAKED POLENTA*

Take the mush above, let cool and slice. Place slices in a buttered dish, dot with butter and rich cheese, add more slices, more butter and more cheese till the dish is full. Bake until the top is brown.

*CORN VINEGAR*

Take ripe corn and soak it overnight in twenty times its volume of water. Heat gently till it starts to swell. Don't let it burst. Strain off the cooled liquid and add four cups of sugar or honey for every kilo of corn. Leave the liquid in the sun in a bottle without a lid. It should become vinegar in about a month. Heat to boiling, take off the heat, bottle and seal.

*HOMINY*

Boil your corn or maize kernels till they are slushy – corn needs less cooking than maize, and young maize needs less than old. Add a teaspoon of salt to every three cups of slush (it should be dry enough so that no liquid runs out if the pan is tilted). Place in a sealed jar in the fridge or a cool cupboard.

This keeps for months. When you want to serve it, heat it up, add butter to taste, with perhaps cream and sugar. It can also be left cold, patted into thin cakes and fried.

# *lettuce*

*Lettuce delighteth to grow in manured, fat, moist and dunged ground: it must be sowen in faire weather in places where there is plenty of water . . . and prospereth if sowen very thin.*
PALLADIUS

***If you can grow*** lettuce ***you can grow*** endive, silver beet, spinach ***and most other*** 'greens'.

## *ROOTS*

Lettuce is easy to grow. In fact, lettuce was once a wild herb springing up along the banks of the Nile after its annual flood. It was probably first cultivated in Central Asia, Kashmir or Siberia, and was being cultivated in China by the 7th century BC.

Good lettuce is much harder to grow. (That original wild lettuce happily seeding itself among the pyramids was tough and bitter.)

Lettuce was eaten both raw and cooked – the cooking probably removed a lot of the bitterness. It was also used medicinally 'they extract its juice at the time of the wheat harvest [autumn, when it would be going to seed and turn bitter], and it is said that it purges away dropsy and takes away dimness of sight and removes ulcers on the eye.' (Theophrastus, 320 BC)

Lettuce was also used to soothe unwanted lust. When Adonis died Venus flung herself into a bed of lettuce to soothe her passion. The medieval herbalist Nicholas Culpepper recommended even more interesting ways to use lettuce to soothe unwelcome amorousness.

## *LETTUCE AND HEALTH*

*The juice mixed or boiled with oil of roses, applied to the forehead and temples, procures sleep, and cured the headache proceeding from a hot cause..*

NICHOLAS CULPEPPER

A diet high in lettuce has been associated with lower rates of lung, stomach and endometrial cancer – the darker green lettuces are best.

Lettuce stalks have been used as a mild soporific – munch them before you go to sleep. (Beatrix Potter's baby rabbits ate lettuce and fell asleep – but you need to be a baby rabbit before eating a salad will make you drowsy.) The milky juice from the stem as it goes to seed has also been used as a sedative and pain reliever, rather like opium, but (hopefully) not addictive.

The medieval herbalist Culpepper recommended lettuce to dampen lust – either eaten or applied directly. If you try this it is a good idea to mention to your partner exactly why you are doing it or they may get the wrong idea.

Eating lettuce seeds was also supposed to make a man sterile. This is probably not a reliable form of contraception.

## *LETTUCE VARIETIES*

Lettuce can be 'hearting' types – like the crisp hearted Iceberg lettuce found in supermarkets, or the softer hearted lettuce like Buttercrunch and Mignonette.

There are also cylindrical lettuces like Cos or Red Cos or Rabbit's Ear. My favourite lettuce are the loose leaf perpetual or continuous lettuce, like Oak Leaf or Perpetual – often with frills like 19th century opera singers' knickers.

There are dozens of lettuce varieties around – summer and winter varieties as well as all year rounders, frilly ones, curly leafed ones, crisp hearted lettuce and broad leafed tougher ones. Try them all. Lettuce has as great a range of tastes as apples.

Most lettuces grow best in either winter or summer. (You can buy Icebergs in the shops all year round because they are shipped from all over Australia.)

Some lettuce can be grown all year round. We grow red and green Mignonette lettuces all year round. They are small – one meal's worth – and sweet, and take both frost and extreme heat. Cos, either red or green, is another all year rounder, and is an excellent lettuce for just picking off the occasional leaf as you need it. Cos lettuce doesn't heart, and the leaves are tougher than most commercial lettuce.

Great Lakes is a common summer lettuce – sweet and crisp. Narrowmar stands hot weather well; Green Velvet and Winterlake are Iceberg types that grow slowly through the winter months. There are dozens more around.

In very hot weather I find that the red lettuces survive better, especially Red Salad Bowl lettuce – a mound of frills, and wonderful to pick leaf by leaf.

Winter lettuce have thicker leaves than summer lettuce. They aren't as sweet either, though they have a more pronounced lettuce flavour. There are several winter lettuce available that look like the summer Iceberg, just tougher.

You can now buy punnets of mixed lettuce – very good value. You can also buy packets of 'mesclun mix' seed, which will give you a mix of delicious and ornamental leaves for salads, including lettuce, rocket, endive and others.

Lettuce seed keeps for at least three years, so it's fun to buy several varieties of seed at once, and plant a pinch of each of them.

## *CULTIVATION*

### *Why you should grow your own*

Lettuce may be treated with Mancozeb, Maneb or Zineb every 7 to 10 days for mildew. These are all dithiocarbamates, possibly carcinogenic and teratogenic. A residue of the dithiocarbamates, ethylene thiourea, stays on the skin even after it's been washed or cooked. Lettuce may also be polluted with endosulphan – this has possibly delayed effects on human health and is extremely harmful to birds, earthworms and other animal life.

### *Essential information*

Feed and water well, and generally don't offend your lettuce or it will turn bitter. Plant the right variety for your climate and time of year.

### *Keeping lettuce seed*

This is easy. If you grow Mignonettes that grow all year round, just let a lettuce go to seed and sprinkle its seeds on the ground – then plant out the seedlings.

Lettuce are self-pollinating, but if you grow any other variety nearby that flowers at the same time, you may get some crossing. Don't collect lettuce from the first plant that goes to seed – its kids may go to seed early too. Choose the best lettuce you have, stake it as it goes to seed (so it doesn't fall over in a storm). Then, when it's finished flowering, pull it up roots and all, and hang it up in a shady, airy spot and catch the seed as it ripens. Or just leave the whole plant in the garden and gather what you can – the first seed to ripen is usually the best.

I don't bother cleaning the chaff off my lettuce seed – just make sure it's all quite dry and leave it in an envelope in a dark, dry place. Use it all next season if you can or the season after. After that, many of the seeds may not germinate, and after five years or so none will.

### *Sowing*

Lettuce is an annual. It can be planted at any time of the year – just choose a winter or summer or all year round variety. Lettuce won't grow in cold weather, though, so if your ground is too cold to sit on comfortably your lettuce will just sit there sulking, then go to seed as soon as it warms up.

I usually stop planting in late autumn, and start again in spring. In frost free areas lettuce keep growing all year. In very hot areas lettuce is best grown in semi-shade or under a shade cloth in the worst of the heat. Lettuce is really a cool season crop, but luckily many heat resistant cultivars have been specially bred for Australian conditions. Read the back of seed packets, or trust that your local garden centre knows what it's doing with the varieties it is selling for your area.

### *Germination and yield*

*Temperature range* 7-24°C, but prefers temperatures over 16°C.
*Seedlings emerge* 6 to 10 days.
*Time until first picking* Matures in 6 to 12 weeks, depending on variety and how big you want the leaves. Of course, with a lot of lettuce varieties you can pick leaf by leaf from the moment they are big enough to bother with.
*Number of plants needed for a family of four* Plant 12 to 36 non-hearting oak leaf lettuce to pull a few leaves every day. (In cool areas they won't grow much – if at all – in winter, so you'll need to grow twice as many as in a subtropical climate.)

Plant twelve lettuces every two weeks so you have continuously maturing lettuces to eat nearly every night.

In cool areas plant fifty or sixty lettuces to mature for winter and spring eating.
*Number of sowings* Plant lettuces every two or three weeks for continuous crops, or oak leaf lettuces once a year.

### *Growing*

Lettuce wreaks a terrible revenge on anyone who neglects it. It becomes bitter if its growth is checked in any way – or else it bolts to seed. Too little water, too little feeding or too hot a summer all can contribute to lettuce failure.

Lettuce growing just needs organisation. Anyone with a plot of ground (or a dozen or so pots) can pick their own lettuce whenever they need it – as long as they remember to feed and water it regularly and pick it when it's ready.

### *Planting*

You can either plant lettuce seed or buy seedlings. One pinch of lettuce seed will give you almost enough lettuces to feed Australia. Beware – it is very easy to overplant lettuce and very hard to harden your heart and pull up the ones you don't want. (Turn them into lettuce soup – see page 83.) I often buy punnets – there are some very good ones that give you a wide range of lettuces that mature at different times. I also like to plant seed of unusual lettuces – but then, we eat a lot of lettuce. Lettuce seed can either be sown in a pot and transplanted, or scattered in place and the ones you don't want thinned out. In hot weather it's best to sow them where they are to be grown, as transplanting can cause them to go bitter. (I warned you – lettuce is temperamental!) If you do transplant in hot weather, cut the tops off to reduce transpiration and loss of moisture. Don't worry – more leaves will grow back.

Keep the soil moist, either with a very thin scattering of sawdust, very fine grass clippings, or even by spreading shade cloth over it to stop a hard crust forming.

Lettuce seeds may not germinate over 30°C. Don't panic. Spread the seeds on wet blotting paper, cover with another sheet of wet blotting paper and keep them in a plastic bag in the fridge for two or three days, then scrape them carefully onto the soil, cover and keep moist.

Plant a few seedlings regularly. It's tempting to plant lots of lettuce seedlings at once – then you end up with a bumper crop for two weeks and none afterwards. Stagger your lettuce plantings.

Lettuce doesn't like competition. Make sure the soil is well weeded and there aren't other plants crowding it. If lettuce is too crowded it may grow slowly (and become bitter), and too much humidity will turn the lettuce slimy. On the other hand, lettuce do seem to like being crowded together – just not with other plants – and are sweeter and more tender if they are shoulder to shoulder with their friends. I plant lettuce about as far apart as the width of my hand.

Keep lettuce seedlings mulched. This will keep the soil cool and moist and help feed them. Well mulched lettuce are much less likely to turn bitter or 'bolt' to seed.

Water every second day – or every day in hot weather, preferably in the evening: hot, wet lettuce may rot.

### *Feeding*

Lettuce have shallow roots, which means they need excellent feeding and frequent watering if they're not to be 'set back' and turn bitter.

Lettuce is best *very* well mulched and fed every week with home-made liquid fertiliser, rich in all sorts of things, not just nitrogen. As it's so shallow rooted it can be planted with good results in a very shallow trench of compost. Avoid using fresh, raw manure – it may cause puffiness and also appears to attract pests to lettuce. Old cow manure or wilted comfrey make excellent mulches for lettuce.

A good way to grow lettuce is to dig a small, shallow trench about half a finger deep and plant your seedlings. Then, as they grow, fill in the trench with compost or sieved old manure. If you don't have compost then feed your seedlings with a sprinkle of blood and bone or old hen manure – say 2 kg per thirty metres of lettuce row.

You can also feed lettuce every week with liquid manure – either home-made or a commercial variety (there are several good ones on the market). I cover weeds with water in a bucket with a lid and add either a little blood and bone, hen manure or fresh urine. Scoop off the liquid and water well. Another easy liquid manure is made by covering compost with water. Compost water is also good to combat rotting lettuce.

If your soil is very acid, a gentle sprinkle of lime or dolomite will help your lettuces flourish. Wood ash will add potash as well as neutralising the soil. Sprinkle gently as though you were sieving icing sugar onto a cake.

Lettuce tolerates acidic to alkaline soil.

### *A box of lettuce*

One styrofoam box filled with lettuce will give you enough lettuce for one person four times a week.

Fill your box with compost or potting mix. Make sure there are holes in the bottom, or the box will fill with water, the soil will turn sour and the lettuce roots will rot.

Choose a non-hearting lettuce variety like Cos or Red Cos or Salad Bowl lettuce, so you can pick a few leaves whenever you want them. Plant the seedlings about a handspan apart. (They won't grow very big because you are going to keep on picking them.)

Now start feeding. Give a little diluted liquid manure once a week. The small amount of soil in a styrofoam box can't possibly hold all the nutrients your plants will need – so you'll have to keep adding them regularly in small amounts. Water every day too – remember, if you treat your lettuce badly it'll turn bitter.

## *COMPANION PLANTING FOR LETTUCE*

Lettuce seem to grow best in mid-summer in the semi-shade of climbing beans or corn. Tomatoes may shade them, but lettuce seem more prone to mildew next to tomatoes.

Lettuce grows very well with celery. Both need massive amounts of water and food and the celery will partially shade the lettuce, while the shallow rooted lettuce won't compete with the deeper rooted celery.

## *GROWING PAINS*

### *Bitter lettuce*

Lettuce that have had any check in their growth may become bitter. Keep your lettuce well watered and well fed. Mulch heavily in hot weather.

### *Lettuce that race to seed*

These will have thick central stalks and no hearts. Lettuce seedlings may appear to transplant well, but then run to seed prematurely. If you are transplanting large seedlings in hot weather, cut off two thirds of their tops to cut down moisture loss. In hot weather, keep a sprinkler on them during the heat of the day for a few days. Use bolt resistant varieties like Narromar, Red Mignonette and Great Lakes.

### *Slugs and snails*

No, you haven't lost your memory. You really *did* plant those lettuce seedlings yesterday. The slugs and snails ate them all last night!

Slugs and snails love lettuce. They'll also crawl into the outside leaves of mature lettuce and although slugs and snails taste better with salad dressing, they don't improve the texture. Wash mature lettuce well – or at least check for wild life. Place snail pellets in old margarine containers with a little door cut out. The snails will eat the pellet and die – but other creatures like dogs, cats, kids and worms won't be annihilated as well.

***Slimy lettuce***

This is caused by too much overhead watering. Mulch. This will keep soil moist and prevent contact between the lettuce and the soil so that soil pathogens are not washed up onto the leaves during watering.

***Lettuce that fail to heart***

Some lettuce never heart – don't expect a Cos lettuce to look like a supermarket Iceberg. Lettuce can also fail to heart if you've fed them too much nitrogen and water at the expense of other necessary elements, especially during hot weather. Avoid artificial, nitrogen-rich fertiliser. Mulch well.

***Big veined lettuce***

This is a virus. Dig plants out and burn them. Only use seed from healthy plants. Practice crop rotation.

***Aphids***

These small, green, clustered insects can be squashed by running your fingers over them. Other aphids will avoid the cemeteries of their brethren. Alternatively, cover marigolds with boiling water, cool, strain and spray. Marigold spray kills and deters aphids.

***Downy mildew***

This shows as pale to darker brown spots on the leaves. Avoid overhead watering, mulch to stop splashing spores, and spray with seaweed spray as a preventative measure. Badly infected plants should be pulled out, as they will probably never be appetising. Compost fed plants are much more resistant.

## *FROM THE GARDEN TO THE TABLE*

***The harvest***

*Fresh eating period* All year with planning – Red Mignonette can be harvested all year round, but won't grow much in cold weather.
*Storage time* At least a week in the fridge. Lettuce purée can be frozen and used for soup.

*Food value* 76 kj per 100 g, vitamins A and C, potassium and thiamin.

### *Picking lettuce*

Non-hearting lettuces like Cos can be picked leaf by leaf, as you need them. Other lettuces may regrow if you slice them off at the roots, but – except in cool weather – the regrowth is usually bitter. I pull our lettuce out by the roots, then plant another seedling straight away.

Most lettuce goes limp soon after picking. Pick it just before you need it, or keep it in the fridge. Don't soak lettuce to recrisp it – it will lose vitamins and flavour. I prefer not to wash lettuce – just wipe it with a damp tea towel. No matter how well you drain a washed lettuce, some water remains – and wet lettuce means a soggy salad.

#### *LETTUCE SALAD*

Like bread, rice and other basics, a lèttuce salad can be wonderful – or horrible.

Firstly, make sure the lettuce is fresh. It must also be dry – either drain it well or, better still, just wipe it with a damp cloth instead of rinsing it. Never soak lettuce – if it is limp, try putting it in the fridge to crisp it, not in water.

Mix in the dressing at the last minute, or it'll go soggy. Don't beat a lettuce salad like a cake – the most gentle mixing possible is best, either with a broad spoon or even with your hands.

#### *LETTUCE AND CROUTON SALAD*

Take large chunks of very fresh french bread. Toast it very lightly. The outside should be crisp while the inside is soft. Dress your lettuce salad, then add the toasted bread chunks at the last minute. Serve at once. The light toasting will help stop the dressing soaking into the bread (as long as the lettuce isn't swimming in vinaigrette).

Thin slivers of cold chicken mixed into this salad also go well with the bread.

*LETTUCE SOUP*

This is good when you want to use up all those lettuce seedlings you planted too lavishly or if you're a canny soul and just can't bear to waste the outside leaves and don't have a rabbit.

Simmer one cup of lettuce (I know it's hard to judge this but the exact proportions don't matter) in three cups of chicken stock for five minutes or thereabouts. Purée. Heat again or chill. Serve with a splash of cream or light sour cream and maybe a sprinkle of well chopped parsley, a little winter or summer savoury, or fresh dill.

*FLAVOURING PEAS*

Add a few lettuce leaves (the outside ones will do) to your peas as you boil them – it accentuates the flavour.

# *onions*

*An honest laborious country man with good bread, salt, and a little parsley, will make a contented meal with a roasted onion.*
EVELYN, ACETARIA, 1699

### *ROOTS*

Onions probably originated in Southern Russia and the Middle East. They were disseminated by just about everyone, from the primaeval Indo-european hordes to the Romans, all of whom took their favourite varieties with them. The ancient Egyptians worshipped the onion, as well as cats and garlic: hardy creatures all of them.

### *ONIONS AND HEALTH*

Onions are high in sulphur – said to be good for those prone to pimples or eczema, and with mucous problems in nose, sinuses, chest, etc. A cut onion used to be left in the sickroom to absorb the foul odours that caused the illness – don't rely on it.

Eating onions – and taking onion cough syrup made by soaking chopped onions in honey – used to be a remedy for asthma and respiratory disease. Onions may also act as an anti-inflammatory drug similiar to prednisolone. (You need to use raw onions for this – unfortunately at least one a day!) Onions (or the quercetin in onions) may also have anti-histamine effects for asthma, hay fever and eczema. Onion juice also destroys a range of bacteria. (Note that many plants and extracts are antibacterial. But, fortunately, few kill all or even most bacteria as, quite possibly, they aren't the ones you want dead.)

According to a Chinese study (National Cancer Institute,

Shandong Province) the more garlic and onions eaten, the lower the risk of stomach cancer – one onion a day reduced the chances of stomach cancer by 540 per cent.

Eating raw (or very lightly cooked) onions may boost high-density lipoprotein levels in your blood. This may help reduce the low- density lipoproteins and control cholesterol levels. Eating onions is a traditional remedy for lowering blood pressure and reducing blood clotting tendencies.

My own tests indicate that onions are an effective insect repellent. The same tests showed quite clearly why no one in their right mind would want to use onions on their skin to repel pests. (To be honest I'm not quite sure why I tested them.)

### *ONION VARIETIES*

Onions vary as much as apples – not just the red, brown and white ones we are used to in shops. Some are so mild and sweet you can chomp them like a peach – they are also reputed to be milder if grown in hot, dry conditions.

If you're growing your own it's a pity to stick to the conventional varieties – though even these will be infinitely more interesting if they are home-grown.

Generally, white varieties – especially the flat white ones – and red ones should be used in the first six months after picking; brown onions keep longer. Pukehoe is a sweet, brown onion with superb storage qualities. Alisia Craig is enormous but doesn't keep quite so well.

Early Barletta is one of the earliest. Hunter River Brown is an early brown. I love Odourless – a mid-season flat whiteish brown, with mild creamy flesh – very sweet and full of flavour. Red Skin is another good mid-season and not a bad keeper. White Imperial and Brown Spanish are good, long-keeping late onions.

Note that all onions can be used as spring onions – just pick the tops off when they're young – but plant proper spring onions or shallots (quite a different flavour) if you want to use them regularly throughout the year. They are also perennial, so they can be cropped forever – just keep feeding and watering them. We use masses of spring onions – they're a good standby when you've used up the last of the onion harvest.

Potato (multiplier) and tree (Egyptian) onions grow from small sets of bulbs planted in autumn. Bulbs form below ground and on top of the stem. They're good and fun and easy to grow – but I find them too fiddly to bother with in large numbers.

## *CULTIVATION*

Onions were one of the last things I learnt to grow for myself. After all, why bother? Onions are cheap, store well, every local shop has them and they don't have the subtlety of flavour that you get in other home-grown vegetables.

Except I was wrong. The first home-grown onion I ate was a revelation. I learnt why many peasant cultures eat raw onion, with maybe a tomato in the other hand and a slab of bread . . . Home-grown onions are sweet and have flavour as well as being acrid. They add richness to anything you use them with. Once you get the hang of it they are easy to grow – and one of the few things you can plant in winter. (Apart from rhubarb and asparagus crowns, artichokes and other spring delicacies . . . but they're not the subject of this book . . .)

Onions are arguably the world's most popular vegetable, and have been for millennia. Travellers seemed to have only needed to sniff an onion to decide it needed to be taken back to their homeland. You find recipes with onions in China, India, the Middle East, Africa, Polynesia (though the latter may be a relatively recent addition to classic recipes). I don't think the Inuit used onions pre-white invasion; but they've perhaps got the only cuisine that's onionless.

Onions can be eaten fresh (they taste much better fresh) but, most importantly during pre-refrigeration times, they store for nearly a year. They also survive cold soil – in medieval England onions were one of the first spring vegetables – the castle celebrated with the first taste of onions after winter (pulled long before fat maturity), knowing that spring greens weren't far behind.

### *Saving onion seed*

Onion seed is simple to collect. Just leave the best few onions in the ground, and the second year they will go to flower (onion flowers attract a vast range of insect predators that will help control the pests in your garden) and then to seed. It's best to stake onions going to seed – they get tall and top heavy, and are inclined to fall over when you least expect it. Pick the seeds when the stalk turns brown and the seeds black and the first few seeds start popping out of their cases. Stick a paper bag over the head to catch the rest – they may keep ripening and dropping for several weeks. Don't worry of you collect seed capsules and other debris – just make sure that the seeds are dry, and store them in a *cool* dry place.

Onion seeds can last for up to five years (maybe more – I've only kept mine for five years), but in hot humid areas they may only last a year or so – less if they get hot or moist.

You can also take a healthy looking onion, not squishy in the centre, and plant with the pointed side upwards and just poking out of the soil. Wait. Two times out of three it will start to sprout again (if it hasn't been artificially treated to stop sprouting). These sprouts will eventually go to seed and the seed can be harvested.

As onions are pollinated by insects, if you have more than one sort setting seed you may get an interesting cross. This doesn't mean you can only grow one sort of onion – just that you should only let one variety go to seed every year.

### *Germination and yield*

*Seedlings emerge* 2 weeks.

*Time to picking* 3 to 6 months, depending on climate, variety and sowing time, and whether you have the patience to wait till they get enormous.

*How many onions for a family of four* How long is a piece of string? Count how many onions you use each week. Multiply by fifty two – then double or triple, as home-grown onions are so good you'll use masses more. As a rule of thumb, I've never met *anyone* who grew too many onions – unless they were growing them commercially.

### *Planting*

Different onions need to be planted at different times: early ones early, late ones late, etc. – a reasonably simple system. Look at directions on the packet or just trust that the ones you buy are timed properly for your area. We sow a succession of onions to get a succession of onion crops too, from mid-spring through to mid- summer – and hopefully this last lot will keep till the next crop next year. (Late onions are usually, but by no means always, the best keepers. I've found home-grown flat whites last for nearly a year as well.)

Sow direct or transplant from sets bought at nurseries.

*Tropical and subtropical areas* February to May
*Temperate areas* March to July
*Cool areas* April to August

### *Where to grow onions*

Anywhere that's weed free. Onions need full sun, though in hotter areas they'll grow in semi-shade. If they are too shady though, you'll get lush tops and no bottoms – which may not matter. We use a lot of onion tops.

Never plant onions where organic matter like mulch or manure has been dug in – the onions may rot.

### *Growing*

Don't plant onion seedlings too deeply – they may rot. Just cover the white stem base. Water seedlings or seeds in gently – they are easily disturbed. (If you get a violent storm in the next fortnight or so you may have to coax them upright again.)

Onions are slow growing and easily smothered by weeds. If the area isn't weed free the weeds will grow faster than the onions, and by the time spring comes you'll just have weeds. Like carrots, onions don't need to grow in dug soil – they'll force their own way down, but the soil *must* be bare.

The simplest way for the onion novice is to fill a styrofoam box with potting mix and grow your onions in that. At least this way you'll get the hang of growing onions without battling the weeds.

You can also pull up a piece of weed mat where you grew capsicums, etc. last season, and grow onions in the weed free area there (my method).

The dedicated, masochistic gardener of course digs the bed, waters it, waits a month, digs it again then plants the onions and weeds every two weeks after that.

Last century, a popular European way of growing onions was to scatter the seed on smooth bare ground and cover with decayed leaf mould or, even better, decomposed grape skins from the wine harvest. The onions were thinned as they grew, but apparently needed no other care – except watering in dry years.

If your soil is still full of weed seeds and you can't be bothered getting rid of them, plant onions anyway. But **mulch them**, *mulch them*, MULCH THEM to keep the weeds down – or grow them with pansies.

### *Keeping onions weed free*

#### *Onions under the rubbish heap*

Push along last year's heap of old corn stalks and melon vines. Plant the onions in the bare weedless ground below. As the onions grow, use material from the rubbish heap to mulch them.

#### *Onions and clear plastic*

If you like bare ground make it weed free for onions by covering it with *clear* (not black) plastic for three weeks. This will germinate weed seeds then kill them in the hot, wet, airless area under the plastic. Mulch the onions to stop stray seeds from blowing in and germinating.

#### *Onions and pansies*

I discovered this a few years ago. Just plant pansy seedlings with your onions, *thickly*. The pansies cover the ground and so prevent weeds from germinating. But as they are lower than onions they don't crowd them out. I found I got twice as many onions (by weight) in the onion and pansy bed as I did in the weeded, only-onions bed (and almost no onions in the unweeded, only-onions bed).

I've tried other flowers with onions since: snapdragons, calendula, heartsease lupins, marigolds and a few others. All helped keep the weeds down a bit but not as wel as the pansies;

except the marigolds, which helped keep the weeds down but kept the onions down too. Pansies seem best.

### *Feeding*

If onions have been planted in fertile, weed free soil they don't need much attention till you pick them. Unfortunately this onion utopia is rarely found. If weeds spring up – or even if they don't – mulch onions well with a good quality mulch like compost, old leaves or lucerne hay, or even wilted grass clippings. As these mulches break down, they'll also help feed the onions. Don't be tempted to boost them with fertiliser – you'll get spectacular tops and tiny bulbs – if any – and the bottoms may rot as well. Stick to mulch. An exception to this rule is where the soil is so poor that the tops look yellow and stunted from starvation. There I give a single feed with old hen manure, etc. in early spring before the bulbs have started to develop. In this case a feed does do some good – it promotes healthy tops, so big bottoms can grow. You can also get away with a sprinkle of hen manure or other fertiliser at planting – as long as you don't overdo it. Just don't be tempted to bung on some more when the bulbs are growing. You'll regret it!

## *GROWING PAINS*

### *Weeds*

See above.

### *Bolting to seed*

You may have planted the wrong sort. Onions are very dependent on climate, so you need one suited to your area.

### *Onion neck rot*

Avoid decomposed organic matter in the soil – keep it on top and let the worms pull it down.

### *Thrips*

These horrible little pale-yellow to dark-grey things suck the joy out of the onions. Run your fingers over them to squash them.

This will also deter the others. (Who likes feasting in a morgue?) Alternatively, you can wash them off with a strong hose *every day* or spray with derris spray (just add water to the dust) or pyrethrum. The pests are easily killed.

## *FROM THE GARDEN TO THE TABLE*

*Don't weep for me, onion-peeler*
(with apologies to Evita and Andrew Lloyd Webber)

Onions make you cry because they are sulphurous – and as you peel them you are literally squirting dilute sulphuric acid in your eye. Some onions are much more sulphurous – and squirty – than others.

You can peel onions under a cold tap; or chill them first so they're not as juicy; or just hold the onion at arm's length; or peel swiftly but leave the base alone till the last minute – it's the most pungent.

A blind friend used to be given the task of chopping onions at the P & C barbecue at the local show. She could peel them with her eyes shut.

Crying with onions can be very cathartic – a good way to get you bawling if you feel you'd be all the better for a good cry!

### *When to pick your onions*

Onions are ready when the tops are dry. Pull them up and leave them in the sun for a few days to harden and for the heat and sunlight to kill any fungi spores.

### *Storing onions*

Choose the best bulbs with no blemishes. Rub off any loose bits of skin and snip off the tops. Plait them together and hang them in a dark, airy shed or even in the kitchen if you're going to use them soon. (Kitchens are really too moist and steamy to preserve onions for long – but they look good up on the wall for a couple of months.)

The best way to store them is hung up in a string bag or porous basket in a dark larder. Otherwise, bung them in the back of the cupboard but make sure it is well ventilated. Just don't store onions in a damp, stuffy place or you'll end up with onion-flavoured slime.

### *How to chop an onion*

Take a sharp knife – not serrated – with a pointed tip, if possible. Cut the onion down the middle. Place the halves side by side on a chopping board, cut side down. Place the tip of the knife in front of the onion halves and lift the handle, then press down rapidly in a series of cuts across the onion one way, then the other way. This sounds complicated, but once you get the knife in your hand you'll see what I mean. This gives good, small onion pieces.

### *Freezing onions*

Onions store so well fresh, the only reason to freeze them is if you have chopped too many. Freeze the chopped onions as fast as you can – only do a small amount at a time in an uncrowded freezer. They'll be a bit limp, but good for cooking. Or better still, sauté them in olive oil first, then freeze.

### *ONION SOUP*

This was made for us in France about twenty years ago. I was amazed when I watched our hostess whip it up – it took 15 minutes and the ingredients weren't exactly appetising: bread, onions, water and a little oil. But it tasted wonderful. I sometimes make it with stock instead of water, but it doesn't really need it if (and this is a big if) you have good onions, good bread, and rich olive oil.

8 large onions
3 dessertspoons olive oil
4 cups water
4 slices good white bread (*not* Tip Top's best)

You can make it at a pinch with wholemeal but it's not as good. Rye bread though makes a lovely soup – but very different from the delicate taste you get with white bread.

Peel and chop the onions. Sauté them as slowly as you can in the olive oil till they turn gold – not black or dark brown, just that slow, rich golden colour that comes from long, long cooking.

Crumble the bread and add it to the oil, and cook that too till it *just* turns colour.

Add the water. Bubble for five minutes. Serve hot. The soup will be pale brown and slightly thick and glutinous. You can scatter on chopped spring onions if you like.

*BAKED ONION IN CREAM*

Chop onions. Cover with cream. Bake until the onions are soft and the top is golden – wonderful!

# *peas*

*Good peason and leekes, to make a poredge in Lent*
*And peascods in July, save fish to be spent.*
*These baviung, with other things, plentifull then*
*Thou winnest the love of labouring men.*
THOMAS TUSSER, *Five Hundreth Pointes of Good Husbandrie*, 1573

***If you can grow one kind of pea, you can grow others, like*** snow peas, mangetout peas, dried peas

### *ROOTS*

Peas are an ancient crop, grown throughout Europe, Asia Minor and China as far back as the days of Homer. They were one of the staple foods of medieval Europe mostly eaten dried and recooked as pease pudding: 'pease pudding hot, pease pudding cold, pease pudding in the pot, nine days old'. Another version calls it pease porridge.

Fresh peas gained popularity under Henry VIII and Elizabeth I, great gourmets (the love of food often goes with great intelligence) although dried peas are still used for such glories as pea sauce and pea and ham soup. Don't condemn dried peas if you've only eaten today's tasteless packaged things. If you dry your own, you'll find they are sweet and good – as different as your own fresh peas will be from commercial rubbery ones.

### *MEDICINAL PEAS*

Peas are said to lower the blood cholesterol level. They are a good source of protein in vegetarian and low meat diets, and excellent for diabetics and those with hyperglycaemia.

### *PEA VARIETIES*

I prefer climbing peas as the short varieties still tend to collapse – and who wants to crouch down to harvest them?

***Bounty***
A short variety, with masses of peas and able to withstand humidity and heat – very resistant to powdery mildew. A good pea to grow where others won't.

***Greenfeast***
A popular variety, one metre tall.

***Novella***
A leafless pea, short variety, resistant to powdery mildew.

***William Massey/ Melbourne Market***
A fast maturing early pea.

***Roi de Carouby***
A delicious French climbing variety with purple flowers. Purple flowered peas are usually hardier in cold conditions.

***Snow peas***
These are picked before the seeds begin to form.

***Mammoth sugar***
Two metres of massively cropping vine.

***Snap pea/Mangetout pea***
These are eaten pod and all. Pick them when the pod is well filled, but don't leave them too long.
*Dwarf sugar snap* about 45 cm tall.
*Sugar snap tall* about 2 metres high.

## *CULTIVATION*

### *Why you should grow your own*

*Commercial disadvantages* Peas may be sprayed with endosulphan (see onions) or fenthion. The latter is a persistent organophosphate with a half life of several weeks, very toxic to dogs and, especially, birds. It may inhibit the enzyme cholinesterase necessary for nerve transmissions.

### *Essential information*

Peas are annuals.

*Make sure peas mature when the temperature is under 40°C or they won't set*. Watch out for birds, wallabies and small children who'll eat them raw after school.

Peas are one of the least – and most – rewarding plants to grow. They are rewarding because if you haven't tasted fresh peas you'll be stunned by your first picking. The harvest though will probably be less rewarding – it is amazing how many vines you need for a saucepan full of peas. Snow peas, however, are much more generous – and if you can grow peas you can grow snow peas. Just pick them before the pods fill. The more you pick the more you'll get for at least a month, if not two – it's having to fill all those pods that takes the peas' energy, so you get fewer pea pods with 'straight' peas.

- Make sure peas will mature in cool but frost free weather.
- Choose a sunny, fertile spot – or at least mulch with compost or feed with liquid or quickly soluble fertiliser (like blood and bone or hen manure) in poor soil.
- Choose climbing varieties – peas are best staked anyway, so you may as well get more for your space and grow climbers.
- Stake well.
- Pick regularly – the peas will be smaller, sweeter . . . and you'll get more peas.

*Pea magic*

If you want to know the name of the person you'll marry, find a pea pod with nine peas in it and lay it under the door or on the door lintel. The name of the next person who comes in will be the name of the person you will marry – or else that person will be very like the person you'll marry.

Alternatively you'll marry the first single person – or dark haired man – to come through the door.

### *Keeping pea seed*

Peas are one of the truly foolproof seeds. Just let your peas dry on the vine and choose the biggest, best and earliest or latest maturing. Peas are self pollinating, so they are fairly safe to come true to type. But separate them from other pea varieties, just in case.

Snow peas and mangetout/sugar/snap peas can be treated the same way. Just leave the pods on the vine till they start to look dry and transparent – you'll realise what I mean when you see it happen.

If it's rainy and the peas are mildewing, haul up the vine, soil and all (keep as much soil on the root as you can) and hang the vine under shelter in an airy place. Pick off any flowers and very immature peas, and the rest will keep maturing.

Pea seed will germinate for about 5 to 10 years after picking. Snow pea seed doesn't last as long. Big fat pea seeds last better.

### *Sowing*

*Tropical areas* March to July
*Subtropical areas* March to July
*Temperate areas* February to June. Avoid months with cold days as well as frosty nights, as seed may rot if there isn't enough warmth for it to germinate.
*Cool areas* July to October. (Seed may rot if the soil is very cold or badly drained.) Then late January or early February, as long as it's not a heat wave, for autumn maturing peas.

### *Germination and yield*

*Germination temperatures* 7-24°C, but prefers at least 13°C. Avoid growing peas if the temperature will go above 24°C for more than two hours a day.
*Seedlings emerge* 7 to 10 days.
*Time to maturity* 12 to 16 weeks for dwarf peas; 14 to 16 weeks

for climbing peas; 8 to 10 weeks for snow peas. It depends on warmth and variety. Peas will crop for several months.
*Amount for a family of four* 4 to 6 square metres of dwarf peas for avid pea eaters; a 2 to 4 metre row for climbing peas.
*Successions* Peas crop for several months if well treated. If your season permits a second crop, plant at least a month later.

### *When to plant peas*

Plant peas so they are setting seed in cool weather. If the weather is over 24°C you won't get peas – though you can try growing a hot weather crop under a pergola.

Any pea can be picked as a snow pea before the pods form – but genuine snow peas are tenderest. Try 'snap' peas too – eat them pod and all. Add pea pods to soup for extra flavour; scoop out the pods at the end of cooking.

### *Planting*

Sow pea seeds about 5 cm deep – about as deep as they are wide – and about 2 cm apart. I plant two pea seeds together, so they twine around and help support each other, and if one pea is taken by ants or eaten by snails there'll still be one there.

Climbing peas need a trellis to climb on – the taller the better, as some can ramble up two metres or more. Even dwarf peas do best with some support. I grow our peas two or three deep along a trellis and mulch them well. Once they've clambered up their trellis and are established, they don't need weeding – they grow above the weeds. Trellis-grown peas seem more disease resistant too.

### *Feeding*

Peas need good fertility to thrive, though too much nitrogen will promote leaf at the expense of the peas and may inhibit fruit set. I scatter a handful of dolomite every square metre just before planting. This gives a better crop and probably helps the amount of nitrogen fixed in the soil too.

The old-fashioned technique was to plant peas in rows of trenches filled with compost – about as wide and deep as the length of your thumb. (Or just scatter compost down a row and press the pea seed into it.) The young peas will be given a boost by the compost and you can give them fortnightly doses of liquid manure – preferably plant rather than manure based, and not too high in nitrogen.

If you don't have compost, try mulching the peas well when they first emerge and scattering on any of the quick-fix fertilisers. Don't feed again. By the time they are flowering the 'quick fix' will have been absorbed – or disappeared into the air or ground water – and the slight nitrogen deficiency will mean more pea flowers, better setting, and fewer pests. Peas will tolerate a mildly acidic soil.

I find peas respond best to a loose mulch between rows, like hay or corn stalks instead of grass clippings or leaves. Denser mulches promote stem rots and mildew during wet weather, particularly in cool conditions where evaporation is low and dews may be heavy.

Peas can also be hilled with compost or soil – or mulch – if you have the energy. This will give you a better crop (peas are very susceptible to heat and drought and this insulates their roots and helps keep in moisture), and the peas will be less likely to fall over with wind or the weight of moisture on their leaves after rain or watering. Peas also need ample oxygen in the soil: they do badly on compacted or waterlogged soil, and mulch is a good preventative and cure for both.

## *Other ways of growing peas*

### *Peas on a stake*

Hammer a stake into the grass, top it with an old bicycle wheel, or radiate more stakes out from the top. Plant pea seed in some compost around the stake – three rows deep. Train the peas up the stake then along the spokes, trailing them over and around till they twine thickly over the lot.

### *Trailing peas*

Plant peas in a window box or hanging basket, and let them trail down. I grew snow peas that way this year – it was the only way we could keep the wallabies from eating them and the lyrebirds from digging them up. They cropped for a couple of months.

Three large hanging baskets gave us a meal of snow peas every day – till we got sick of them.

### *Peas as nitrogen fixers*

Peas are nitrogen fixers – or at least the bacteria associated with their roots are: about 80 kg a year   Note that the nitrogen fixed by the peas will only be available after the leaves, stems, etc. have decayed back into the soil. If you are using peas for green manure slash them just as they start to flower, otherwise they will toughen and most of the nutrients go to the peas, not back to the soil. Don't bother digging them in – just use the nitrogen-rich mulch around other crops.

We grow masses of peas – not just as vegies, but as fertiliser and soil conditioner: arches of peas in any 'spare' bit of the vegie garden, or dwarf peas between rows of other veg, sweet peas and perennial sweet peas sprawling all over the place. I reckon a good half of our nitrogen needs are 'fixed' by our pea crops.

## *COMPANION PLANTING WITH PEAS*

Grow climbing peas up old corn stalks, Jerusalem artichoke stems or old sunflower stems, or plant them in a ring of compost around a young deciduous tree that will lose its leaves in early autumn when the peas are flowering.

Peas are excellent crops to grow before other vegetables. I used to grow peas commercially with corn – the peas climbed up the corn and the pea slash fed the next corn crop.

Onions or garlic are a good crop to grow in between pea crops if there has been a problem with pea blight or wilt. Growing peas in a bed of perennial chamomile may help kill mildew spores left in the soil – just push the seeds into the chamomile, mulch them when they emerge and then stake them. The chamomile will grow back when you've pulled out the pea vines.

## *GROWING PAINS*

### *Birds*

Birds like pea seeds and very young pea plants and will eat the peas out of the pod – or even steal the whole pod and fly away with them. Cover the peas with an old mosquito net or bird netting. Spray the plants red with watercolour. Pick peas every day so birds don't get in the habit of feasting there. Grow climbing peas with climbing beans to disguise them both.

***Powdery mildew***

This shows as a powdery covering on the foliage. Stake the peas so air can flow around them. In humid areas angle the rows so the wind flows down them, not across, maximising the area exposed to the wind. Spray with seaweed spray or compost water as a preventative. (Just cover seaweed or compost with water and use when it turns pale brown – keep it covered so mozzies don't breed there and flies can't visit and sip.) In bad cases, use half-strength bordeaux.

Always clean up pea debris – all the old leaves and stalks – after a crop of peas: they will probably be infected and may pass on the early infection to the next crop.

***Empty pods***

This may be due to frost damage. Wait for warmer weather. Hunt for caterpillars and squash them or use Dipel. And don't forget: some birds are pea gourmets (see above).

***Bacterial blight***

The signs are dark brown edges or splodges on the leaves. The stem may also develop splodges, and both the leaves and stem may shrivel.

Don't replant peas for at least three years in an affected area. Use only healthy seed. Collect all infected matter from a crop and burn or hot-compost it. Don't pick or weed peas in wet weather. See also the solutions for powdery mildew.

Compost fed plants are much more resistant, as are plants well mulched with rotting lucerne or wilted comfrey.

***Snails***

Place pellets in old margarine containers with a little door cut out for snails to enter.

### *Ants*

Ants love pea seeds. In cool weather, cover pea seed with old cooking oil and dust with white pepper or ground chilli. Ants don't like their food hot and spicy.

### *Rotting seed*

Cover with old cooking oil, as above. Don't overwater pea seed until the seedlings emerge – it rots easily. Make sure the soil is well drained and there is no undecomposed organic matter in the soil.

## *FROM THE GARDEN TO THE TABLE*

I love peas: peas with roast chicken, fresh pea soup, peas through rice, creamed pea sauce on pasta. I even eat frozen peas if I don't have fresh peas – or even bought peas, bland and leathery after you've grown your own. At least these evoke the memory of real peas – if not the sweetness and the crunch.

There is nothing like fresh peas. If I ever have to choose my final meal it will contain peas – tiny, almost fragrant, rushed from the garden to the pot.

### *Harvest*

*Fresh eating period* About six weeks per crop. Crops best in cool weather – the flowers don't set in heat. Try planting in January and February for autumn peas.

*Storage time* 2 to 3 weeks in the fridge. Can be frozen or dried. If you are freezing peas, dump them in boiling water for one second, then dry them and freeze them. Treat snow peas the same way. Fresh frozen peas taste quite good – better than no peas at all and much better than commercial frozen peas, or commercial fresh peas. Frozen snow peas are rubbery, but not too bad cooked. Just remember that they give out more liquid after freezing, and can make a stir fry a trifle damp. Best added at the last minute and just heated, instead of cooked.

*Food value* 335 kj per 100 g; vitamins A and C; potassium, iron, phosphorus, thiamine, calcium

Peas take about 12 week to mature, though some like Early

Massey will crop faster. If you treat your peas well – and they don't get powdery mildew – you'll be able to keep picking them for at least two months.

Pick peas when the pods are well filled but while the pods are still tender. Older peas don't taste as good. This goes for sugar/ snap/ mangetout peas too – and snow peas should be picked as soon as the white flower drops off the end and they are about a long as half your finger and the peas inside are still pin pricks, not true seeds.

Peas are sweetest and less rubbery if they are picked in the cool of the day – best in the morning, or in the evening after dusk, just before you cook them.

Peas are easily shelled. (A few decades ago women used to carry bags of peas with them, and shell them as they watched an afternoon concert in the park, or had a cup of tea with friends.) If you are going to cook the pea pods, wash them very well if they have been sprayed with fungicide.

*Coping with surplus peas*

Dry them for soup or stews (just leave them in the sun till hard or let them dry in the pod on the vine); grind the dried peas in a flour mill or coffee grinder for pea flour; add it to stews, etc. for thickening, or to bread for flavour and protein. Old-fashioned blue flowered peas used to be the classic ones for drying and grinding into pea flour – but most peas can be dried, though only the blue flowered ones will give a truly fine flour.

*How to cook peas*

Fresh peas need nothing else. *Just* cover with water – no salt – and simmer for five minutes or till tender. The time will vary – very tiny peas (one of the most exquisite things in the world) only take about two minutes.

If your peas are slightly older add some of the pea pods to give more flavour or add a little honey (not sugar – the taste isn't as good). Older peas need longer cooking.

I have to hide our freshly picked peas from my offspring – otherwise they're all eaten raw. Very, very fresh raw peas are delicious – very tender, very sweet.

*Cooking snow peas*

Don't avoid them just because you've tried raw snow peas in salads before and hated them. Snow peas need to be eaten as soon as they're picked or they turn rubbery and very slightly bitter.

Chomp them raw – they are sweet and delicious. Steam them till they turn bright green, then take them off the heat at once – they don't need much cooking. Stir fry them – just toss in hot oil with a bit of garlic or grated fresh ginger. Again, hoick them out when they turn bright green.

*Mangetout peas*

Steam or boil for about ten minutes – the older the peas the longer it will take to make them tender.

*WHOLE PEAS*

This is good for peas that are very slightly past their prime. Cover with hot water, boil for 5 minutes, drain and serve whole on wide plates. You pick up the pods with your fingers and suck out the peas. Peas cooked in their pods are sweeter and more flavourful.

*PEA FLOUR CHAPATIS*

Add water to pea flour, roll out very thinly and fry in very hot oil. Eat hot.

*PEAS IN CREAM*

1 cup peas
1 cup cream
1 egg yolk
nutmeg
black pepper
chopped parsley
2 tablespoons of lemon juice

Just cover peas with cream. Simmer for about ten minutes. The cream will have greatly reduced by now. Add the other ingredients, heat again gently till the sauce thickens more, but don't boil or it may curdle.

*FRESH PEA SOUP*

1 cup peas
3 cups stock
6 lettuce leaves
cream
nutmeg

Simmer peas and lettuce in the stock for ten minutes. Scoop out the lettuce. Purée and serve with a dash of cream and a dust of nutmeg.

Don't use frozen peas or bought peas – if the peas aren't young, sweet and fresh the soup will be bland and boring.

# *potatoes*

### *ROOTS*

Now the third most eaten crop in the world, there are thousands of potato species, both wild and domesticated: blue, red, orange, almost black, yellow, waxy, one almost flat, one quite round, as well as a hairy one that is said to be pest resistant – the poor things don't like the hair.

Potatoes were originally South American, and have been cultivated for about 8000 years. They may at one time have been worshipped. Probably brought to Europe by a Spanish explorer in the 1500s, they were introduced to Ireland by Sir John Hawkins, and then to England by either Sir Walter Raleigh or Sir Francis Drake.

The story goes that when X (whomever it was – sources differ) presented one to Queen Elizabeth I she wasn't impressed. She ate it raw. The rest of Britain wasn't impressed either – partly because of a rumour that eating spuds caused leprosy.

Potatoes gradually spread over most of Europe, but as ornamentals for the pretty blue flowers, not for their tubers. Fairly soon, someone realised that potatoes weren't mentioned in the Bible. And anything not in the Bible had to be sinful; and if it was sinful it was sexy – so potatoes became popular as an aphrodisiac. 'Let the sky rain potatoes,' cried Sir John Falstaff in Shakespeare's *Merry Wives of Windsor* when he wanted to regain his vigour to cope with the Merry Wives.

Potatoes were sold by street vendors; if you wanted to warm your hands you bought a hot potato and ate it cupped in your fingers.If you wanted to warm your passion you ate even more.

By the 1600s potatoes were the staple food of Ireland (no, potatoes weren't the cause of Irish overpopulation), partly because the absentee landlords' agents – who would confiscate anything harvested and stored in the barn – wouldn't demean themselves by digging up spuds left in the field. The failure of the potato crop in the 1840s led to a series of famines and mass emigration. (The absentee landlords and an inept government's policies contributed too. Ireland remained a net food exporter right through the famine!) Australia owes a large number of its early immigrants to the potato.

## *MEDICINAL POTATOES*

About 5 per cent of people with arthritis improve on a solanaceae free diet – so avoid potatoes and tomatoes, capsicum, chillies, eggplant, etc. Potatoes have also been grated, warmed and used as a poultice on arthritic joints. Potato water – made from the starch-rich juice from grated potatoes – has been used to help against diarrhoea, especially in babies. This potato starch also used to be one of the most popular starches for clothes.

### *Potato aphrodisiac*

The British first regarded potatoes as the devil's crop, because they grow from tubers rather than from seed and aren't mentioned in the Bible. Anything not in the Bible had to be sinful, and if it was sinful it had to be sexy. Potatoes were hailed as an aphrodisiac, and were supposed to turn regular potato eaters into hermaphrodites. It took several hundred years for the British to realise that however they ate their potatoes, they had very little effect at all on the libido. They then turned to tomatoes instead. Don't worry about tomatoes in your salad, though, as long as you include lettuce: lettuce was said to dampen passions, just as tomatoes were supposed to inflame them.

## *SOME POTATO VARIETIES*

Perhaps a thousand varieties of potato have been grown at some time or other – black potatoes, blue potatoes, knobby or egg-shaped – far removed from the neat, white-fleshed, smooth, brown or pink- skinned ones we're familiar with. Over four hundred potato varieties are still grown by specialist growers. Unfortunately only a few of these are grown commercially, and those are the ones that travel best, store best, are highly coloured like Pontiacs or are nice and long for commercial chip making.

Even fifty years ago there were dozens of commercial varieties in Australia. Some like Brown's River, a purple skinned variety grown mostly in Tasmania, or the Vicar of Laleham from Victoria, or Duchess of Bucleuch, Early Puritan, General Kitchener, Royal Kidney and other names have now disappeared. Each district grew potatoes that were suited to it, each cook chose them according to the season and the purpose for which they were to be used. Now, potatoes have become standardised – and not for the better!

If you can get hold of rare varieties, try them. There's as much variation in potatoes as there is in apples – but who can tell once they're mashed to a pulp with milk and butter?

New potatoes are just small potatoes, picked before the plants die off. Unless specified they can be any variety at all.

The following are some of the more common shop varieties.

### *Coliban*

Very white fleshed; a good chipper; not so good for salads, unless baked.

### *Desirée*

These are pink skinned, with a pale yellow flesh. They are originally from Holland. They don't mash well, but boil or steam wonderfully, though a lot of the colour fades from the skin. They make excellent salads, either as new potatoes or as old ones.

### *King Edward*

A large white potato, best for baking. King Edwards disintegrate when boiled, so don't. If you must use them for a salad, bake them instead – though they are a bit too grainy for best results.

### *Brownell*

A red skinned Tasmanian variety.

### *Pontiac*
The main pink-skinned potato grown. Beware though – some are artificially coloured to get better prices. Pontiacs boil and steam well, and are excellent for salads.

### *Sebago*
One of the main types grown. I find commercial ones make an awful salad – too soft and grainy. Home-grown ones are firmer and quite good. They are best used reasonably fresh.

## *CULTIVATION*

### *Why you should grow your own*
Potatoes may have been sprayed with Zineb or Maneb or Mancozeb (suspected carcinogens and teratogens) or a similar fungicide for target spot and other similar fungal problems. The residue of these pollutants is not destroyed when the potatoes are cooked. Potatoes may be sprayed with a wide range of pesticides for ladybirds and other pests. There have also been cases where red potatoes like Pontiacs have been artificially coloured.

Potatoes may be treated to stop them sprouting. Maleic hydrazide (MH), nonyl alcohol, 3-chloroisopropyl-N-phenlylcarbamte (CIPC), isopropyl-N-phenylcarbamate (IPPC), methyl napthaleneacetic acid (MENA), and 2,3,4,6, tetra-chlornitrobenzene (TCNB) are commercial sprout inhibitors. CIPC is most commonly used, either as dust, water dip, aerosol or vapour.

The best potato is a fresh one, preferably home-grown. Potatoes go soft and flabby with long storage and some of the vitamins are lost. Soft, flabby potatoes make soft, flabby potato salads – the dressing soaks into the potato flesh, instead of thickly coating the outside.

Most fresh shop-bought potatoes are poor quality anyway – they turn to a grainy mash when boiled, are soft rather than floury when baked, and disintegrate when fried. This is because they have been grown with too much nitrogen. This means larger potatoes – an excellent result when you're being paid by the tonne, but the potatoes tend to be soft and watery, and poorer keepers than those grown in soils that are high in organic matter.

Home-grown potatoes have a flavour. Shop-bought ones usually don't. Like fresh, free-range chicken or blood red tomatoes, we've forgotten the real taste of potatoes – almost nutty, subtle and pervasive.

*The delights of home-grown spuds*

Spuds are easy to grow, quick to harvest – and you get kilos in a very small space. Why on earth then don't more people grow their own?

Partly, I suspect it is because spuds are cheap – or cheapish. It's all too easy to grab a plastic bag of (soft, mushy, greening) spuds – then have them rot away in a dark cupboard as their shoots get longer and longer and their texture even worse.

Bad spuds are a waste of money. You're better off eating rice or pasta, which is what many people do nowadays – spud consumption is declining every year! But a good home-grown spud will save you money. It'll be so good you savour it, eating less meat and other expensive items, and basing your menu around your home-grown spuds instead.

***Essential information***

Potatoes are an annual

Mulch spuds right up to the bottom or even the top leaves – the more you mulch the more roots grow from the stem, and the more roots, the more spuds.

***Potato seed***

'Seed potatoes' are small, disease free potatoes. True 'potato seed', picked after the potato flowers have set, may not be viable and, if it does grow, will take two years to produce good sized spuds. Potato seed is fun to play around with though – you may find that cross pollination gives you a new variety.

It is illegal to plant potatoes that have sprouted in your cupboard. You should use registered, disease-free seed to prevent disease from spreading (usually via aphids that can carry potato virus for many kilometres). In reality this law is frequently broken and is impossible to police. Don't grow non-certified ones in a potato growing area – you may spread disease – and never use potatoes that may have come from diseased plants. Don't use them either if the shoots are long and thin – this is a symptom of a virus infection.

Choosing your seed potato from the supermarket, however, gives you access to gourmet varieties, most of which aren't sold in garden centres as seed potatoes, and even when you can get hold of them, have to be ordered in bulk. Look for waxy yellow potatoes, or white fleshed perfect baking Colibans, pink Desirées, red Pontiacs or even blue-fleshed Peruvian potatoes – look weird, taste great! Go potato hunting. It's worth it once you taste your own.

If you want to grow a new potato variety, try growing the true seed. Pick the fruit when it is ripe (about 6 - 8 weeks from 'setting'), squeeze the seed out of the fruit into a bowl, and cover with water. Leave for a week to ferment, then wash the seeds clean. Keep them in an old envelope till next spring.

Even if you grow only one sort of potato, you may find considerable variation in the potatoes produced. Save the best and keep growing them – or grow several varieties and see what crosses you produce.

Have fun.

***When to sow***

*Tropical areas* Late February to September.

*Subtropical areas* Late January to September.

*Temperate areas* July, August, September. Then late January to February.

*Cool areas* August to December, though you may get away with a January crop.

*Shoots emerge* Anywhere from 6 days to two months, depending on the time of year and variety of the potato.

*Days to maturity* 16 to 20 weeks, depending on variety and time of year. But you can bandicoot spuds from about 4 to 6 weeks on.

*Number of plants needed for a family of four* 60 to 80 plants, but more if you are going to eat more than one serve of spuds a day – and if you've got home-grown spuds you probably will.

### *Growing potatoes*

You get potatoes by planting another potato – a seed potato – or a piece of potato with an 'eye' and letting it grow into a potato bush. Whole potatoes give the plant a better start and probably give you a bigger crop. The potatoes grow underneath: lovely fat tubers on the roots. Forget about the old laborious dig-and-dig-again methods of growing spuds. There are much easier ways of doing it.

Spuds are warm (as opposed to cold or hot) season crops. Spuds are frost sensitive – they survive light frosts but severe frosts will kill them. They also don't like wet and humid weather.

In hot areas avoid growing spuds in the wet season. Though with above-ground beds and a lot of acres you can grow them all year round.

In cool and temperate areas, plant your spuds any time from the beginning of August onwards – or even earlier as long as the ground doesn't freeze to spud depth. (Frozen spuds will rot.) They won't start to shoot though until the weather warms up. Alternatively, wait till spring, when your winter spuds are shooting in the cupboard, and plant them. Don't plant any that look rotten, or that have very long shoots: they will either die when exposed to hot sunlight, or they may be a symptom of virus disease.

Always plant spuds deep enough so that the soil won't wash away and partially uncover them when you water or when you get an unexpected deluge. In very hot, dry areas spuds can be planted about 30 cm deep to shelter them against extremes. In more temperate areas measure your spud, then put about that depth of soil on top of it.

Potato peelings will sometimes sprout in the compost. Transplant them – or let them fill the compost with new tubers.

#### *Conventional potato growing*

Dig your ground well and deeply. Spread either hen manure or blood and bone – spuds need a fair amount of phosphorus but not too much nitrogen or you'll get all leaf and no spud. Plant the potatoes about a hand span deep. As they start to grow 'hill' them so that the stem is covered by soil. You'll get a larger crop this way, as more roots will form from the stem – and the more root, the more potatoes. It also helps stop potato moth from burrowing down.

You can also mulch potatoes with leaves or lucerne hay or well dried lawn clippings etc instead of soil. This gives better results.

*Potatoes in old tyres*

This is my favourite method. Pile one tyre on top of another then pile up more next to that, so you have a bed two deep. Throw a little mulch or compost into the tyres, throw in your spuds, throw in more hay, compost, wilted weeds, etc. Then wait. As the green shoots poke up, throw in more weeds or hay, so that only the top leaves ever show.

When the plants die down just lift the tyres and kick the mulch apart to find your potatoes. Or just wriggle your hand in and pull out what you need and let the rest re-grow.

I find this an excellent method – the black absorbs heat and the potatoes grow even in cool weather, sometimes through most of winter. It does need more watering, though, in dry times.

*Comfrey trench*

Dig a long trench about 100 cm deep. Line it with comfrey, at least six leaves deep. Throw down your seed potatoes, cover with a little soil. As they grow, keep adding soil to the trench, so only the top leaves show. When the top of the trench is reached keep mulching with wilted comfrey leaves, or any good mulch.

This trench method can of course be used without the comfrey, which just adds fertiliser. Sprinkle on soil instead and give the crop a sprinkle of blood and bone or old hen manure a fortnight after the shoots have emerged. The trench method simply replaces 'hilling' – you do the hard work before planting instead of after.

*Above-ground potatoes*

Use the method above, but omit the tyres. Throw the seed potatoes onto the ground – use a patch of lawn or weeds – then pile on hay and keep the leaves almost covered as the plants grow. With this method you don't have the trouble of digging, or of finding old tyres – but in dry or hot years it gives a much smaller crop than the above two methods.

At the end of the potato season you'll have a rich, soft, fairly weed free garden bed to plant your broad beans or other winter crops where there was grass or weeds before.

*Potatoes in a pot*

This is suitable for a doorstep or balcony. Put a couple of holes in an old bucket or an old fruit box. Throw in some potting mix, then the seed potatoes. Cover with mulch or more potting mix. Keep the potatoes covered as they grow in the way described above. When the top dies down, up-end your bucket or box: it should be mostly full of potatoes.

All of these 'above ground' methods depend on good quality mulch to feed the crop. Lucerne hay is best or compost or wilted comfrey. Lawn clippings can be used, but they should be well wilted or they'll heat up. Wilted weeds are good too, as long as they are not too 'woody' – if they are, they'll lack nutrients. Add a sprinkle of blood and bone every two weeks to help the weeds break down and keep the spuds growing well.

*Potatoes in a pile of weeds*

Most gardens have a pile of rotting weeds – sometimes called compost heaps, though they aren't. Compost heaps break down quickly. Try poking seed potatoes into the bottom of the pile. They'll sprout – and the added warmth of decomposing weeds will help their growth. Fish out the tubers when the tops die off.

*Potatoes in the grass.*

Dig a hole just big enough for the potato. Cover it. Surround the hole with newspaper, throw mulch on top. Keep the plant mulched to the top leaves as it grows.

*Growing potatoes all year round in cool areas*

We had massive frosts this year – down to minus 10, which is unusual for our valley. But the potatoes still kept growing.

Not the ones in the soil, of course. They died off by May. These were ones planted in tyres, under the shelter of an avocado tree. I piled up tyres two deep, threw a potato onto the grass, threw down some weeds and left them. They grew by themselves as the weeds gradually rotted into soil and the grass below the potato died. I kept throwing in more weeds to keep them mulched almost to the top of the plant.

The 'winter spuds' were only small – bantam egg sized. But they were welcome with other potatoes in the cupboards beginning to sprout, and they kept us going till the spring crop was ready to bandicoot.

I grow potatoes in tyres in early spring and autumn. The rest of the time they grow faster in the ground – or rather I toss them on the ground and cover them with mulch. The more you mulch potatoes – or hill the soil around them – the more spuds you get. Potatoes form on potato branches – if you cover the branches you get more spuds.

Plant your first potatoes about six weeks before the last frost date – here, that's about the beginning of August. The spuds will take about six weeks to sprout and leaf and are fairly invulnerable to cold till then – unless the ground freezes, in which case they'll rot.

***Feeding your spuds, so they can feed you***

Potatoes can be fed by:

- A green manure crop (this is a nitrogen-fixing crop like peas or beans, slashed as soon as it flowers, so the nitrogen returns to the soil), either before the potato crop or grown between the rows and slashed as it grows for instant mulch.
- Mulch
- Adding fertilisers while the plants are growing.

The first probably gives the best results unless you are using a no-dig method. Nitrogen-fixing green manure makes the best fertiliser. Peas, beans, broad beans or lupins should be planted the autumn before and slashed in late winter just as they start to flower, then dusted with old hen manure or blood and bone or any of the quick-fix fertilisers (as a last resort) to help decomposition.

Potatoes grow best with plenty of decomposed organic matter in the soil, but as potatoes don't start growing and taking up nutrients for some weeks, there is time for the green manure to break down and some of its nutrients to become available for the start of the crop. On the other hand, potatoes take up nutrients fastest in their early growing stages and may need some liquid manure 'starter' to get the best results while you are waiting for the green manure to break down.

Never dig in undecomposed organic matter while the potatoes are growing or for several months beforehand. It can cause the potatoes to rot or become diseased. Always leave it on top of the soil to decompose naturally.

Green manuring can be combined with above-ground growing methods. Slash down your crop of, say, peas; place the potatoes on top of the slash, and cover with old stable tailings, compost or even straw liberally watered with home-made liquid manure. Water again with liquid manure every week till the potatoes start to flower.

Potatoes need slightly acid soil – they are more prone to scab and other diseases in alkaline soils. The vigorous growth in acid soil also means they are slightly less prone to various viruses. If eelworm are a problem, try rye, wheat and oats and eelworm-resistant green manure crops. Potatoes are far less susceptible to potato scab if they are fed with compost.

*Always* mulch well – potato stalks grow more roots if they are covered – and the more roots, the more spuds, and the better the plant is able to feed itself. Lucerne hay and seaweed are excellent potato mulches, but any of the high-nitrogen mulches are good. With some early extra feeding, potatoes can get all the rest of the feeding they need from mulch.

If you aren't using mulch, hill the potatoes with soil and give a good sprinkle of blood and bone or old hen manure at planting, and again every three weeks till after flowering.

Potatoes grown in highly nitrogen-rich soil are watery, often grainy and don't store well. Potatoes need adequate potash for a good long- keeping, mealy potato.

Never dig in manure or green manure around potatoes: it will make them more prone to potato scab and rotting. Never fertilise with fresh manure either: it will encourage scab.

## *GROWING PAINS*

### *Symptoms of mineral deficiencies in potatoes*

Nitrogen deficient potato plants are small and stunted. The leaves are light green to yellow and the plants flower early before proper tuber development.

Phosphorus deficient potatoes have brown to greyish green leaves changing later to reddish purple. They are also smaller and stand more upright than usual. Tuber development is delayed and the crop is much smaller than normal.

Potash deficient plants grow abnormally fast at first. The older leaves develop whitish yellow spots around the edges and then turn brown. The leaves sometimes curl downwards, sometimes split at the edges, then die and fall.

Potash deficiency usually starts to show up in waterlogged spots or where the soil is poor generally. Potatoes grown in potash deficient soil tend to be soggy and yield is greatly reduced.

Calcium deficient leaves are light green, with short, weak stems. Plants may die in bad cases. Calcium deficiency is most likely where the soil is very acid. Try a sprinkle of dolomite at the first symptoms – but avoid over-liming.

Magnesium deficient potato plants have bright yellow young leaves with odd spots of green. The older leaves remain green but with dead areas between the leaves.

### *Green potatoes*

These should be thrown out. Potatoes turn green when exposed to light. They are more likely to turn green in the first few hours after digging. Never leave your potatoes on top of the soil, even for half an hour – bag them straightaway. All potatoes contain solanine, but green potatoes contain possibly poisonous amounts.

Symptoms of solanine poisoning resemble gastro-enteritis. Small quantities probably won't make you ill but it's best to be safe. Save green potatoes for seed and don't eat bitter ones. It is not actually the green bits that make you ill – after all that is just chlorophyll – but the greening alerts you to the fact that the whole tuber has gone into growth mode, which is when it is dangerous.

So don't just cut out the green bits thinking that you are making the rest of the potato wholesome – you've just eaten the canary in the coal mine and it hasn't changed the situation.

Store potatoes in a dark place.

### *Black potatoes*

Potatoes turn black or grey when they are cut. This is ugly but harmless. If your potatoes turn black during cooking it's just a reaction with iron in the water – again, harmless. Add a dash of lemon juice or vinegar to the water if this happens.

### *Rotten potatoes*

These stink. You can cut out the bad bit and eat the rest of the potato, though – the firm part of the potato won't have been affected. Make sure soil is well drained with no undecomposed organic matter in it. Don't plant potatoes where there have been rotten potatoes for five years.

### *Potato moth*

Hill the potatoes or make sure they are mulched to the top of the plant so the moth can't get into the tubers or their stalk.

### *Hard potatoes*

These have been infected with a virus. Use certified seed potatoes and make sure you get rid of all infected potatoes.

### *Ladybirds*

Mulching up to the top leaves will mostly keep them away. Spray with pyrethrum as a last resort.

### *Potato blight*

This is the blight that precipitated mass Irish starvation. Dark brownish spots appear on the leaves which increase in size with a green white mould. Leaves die, and lesions appear on the stems.

Potato blight fungus spores are washed from the leaves to the tubers which then rot. Potato blight can be carried by wind, water or infected plants.

Spray with bordeaux in the early stages to prevent spores

washing to the ground. Spray again if symptoms continue after two weeks. If symptoms appear close to harvest time, slash off the tops and burn or compost them. Then spray the stalks with bordeaux. It is worth doing this and getting a slightly smaller crop than risk losing the lot.

***Potato moth***

The moth burrows in potatoes and these may rot.

Make sure no tubers are exposed to allow the female moth to lay eggs in the potatoes: hill and mulch regularly. A companion crop of broad beans planted just before the potatoes, then slashed as mulch before the potatoes mature, is an excellent control.

***Target spot***

This is more widespread than potato blight, slower acting and later. Small spots appear on the leaves which eventually die off. This happens so slowly that the grower may think the plants are dying naturally. Yield will be much reduced. Spray with bordeaux when symptoms appear and every two weeks from then on.

***Soggy potatoes***

These are lacking in potash. Add potash-rich fertiliser or wood ash to the soil – not too much or the soil may become too alkaline. Mulch with comfrey or good compost.

***Aphids***

Plants may wilt at the tips and die off. Large infestations can lead to premature dying off and reduced yield.

Mulch heavily and aphids will avoid the plants. Try reflective mulch between rows or interplant with marigolds, mustard, or nasturtiums; or plant between wormwood hedges, kept well trimmed. As your soil improves, the aphid problem should vanish except in long cool springs.

Use marigold spray – just cover flowers with boiling water, cool, strain and spray. As a last resort spray with glue spray: one cup of flour, one cup of boiling water, then as much cold water as you need to be able to spray it.

### *Eelworm nematodes*

These are wart-like swellings on the potato skin. Eelworm eggs and their larvae can survive two years in the soil. Plant an eelworm resistant green manure crop like rye, wheat or oats, or plants like sweet corn, onions, caulies and cabbage which can tolerate them.

Encourage earthworms with mulch. They eat eelworm eggs and larvae. Several species of fungi encouraged by high levels of decomposing organic matter trap eelworm in mycelium webs.

In other words – mulch.

### *Potato scab*

This shows as small, brown circular or oval scabby encrustations on the potatoes, wich may be affected under the soil with no sign above.

Plant disease-free tubers. Make sure drainage is good. Scab is most prevalent in wet soils with temperatures below 18°C. Spores can remain active in the soil for 15 years or more. A crop of broad beans before the potatoes are planted, dug in and left to rot before planting, will help inhibit scab. Compost-fed potatoes are far more resistant to scab.

### *Common scab*

This may look like potato scab to begin with, but the scabs gradually cover the entire tuber. No symptoms may appear above ground.

Plant only certified seed. Common scab is introduced on infected tubers. It can also infect beetroot and turnips – these should not be grown anywhere you plan to put next season's spuds.

Common scab is worse in dry, warm conditions and in light sandy soils. Mulch well – to keep in moisture and keep up the humus levels.

Avoid liming your potato bed. Once scab is present, green manure the ground before planting and add plenty of compost to help control it. Compost and most decomposing organic matter probably encourage soil micro-organisms antagonistic to scab.

Make sure the soil is kept moist round the potatoes, particularly when the tubers are forming.

***Rhizoctonia scab***

New shoots rot, foliage is bunched or curled, potatoes have cracks or depressions with brownish black scabby lumps on them.

Rhizoctonia scab is worst in cool, wet weather. Make sure your soil is well mulched and well drained, and your seed is disease free with no blemishes at all. Feed with compost, and mulch with wilted comfrey or nettles or well rotted lucerne hay.

***Potato mosaic, leaf curl***

These are virus diseases carried by aphids from infected plants. The symptoms of both include rolled leaf edges. Plants may die early, with yellow veins in the leaves and possibly mottled spots.

These viruses can't be cured once the plant is infected. Plant disease-free tubers and hope your neighbour's aphids don't carry the disease over the fence. Don't use small tubers with long thin shoots for seed potatoes. They may be infected with leaf roll.

The viruses don't remain in the soil after the tubers and aphids have gone. Crops can be planted in the same soil as long as you are sure no small potatoes remain – and this is difficult.

***Potato gangrene***

Potatoes rot from the inside, with deep rounded depressions on the outside. The smell is horrible, like rotten fish.

Plant only disease-free seed. Try not to damage potatoes when digging up or weeding – potato gangrene only affects injured plants at harvest. Never store potatoes that are injured in any way at all, even by a scrape of the digging fork. Any injury can let fungus spores enter. Make sure storage areas are free of dirt and debris from past crops. Compost or actively rotting mulch may inhibit gangrene spores.

## *FROM THE GARDEN TO THE TABLE*

I love potatoes – baked in the oven, with grated cheese and beetroot and sour cream or bits of bacon or baby spuds boiled in their skins with mayonnaise and chopped apples or chopped with seafood for a hot seafood 'salad'. My grandma's spuds roasted and crisp and so good we only needed one slice of meat to go with our baked potatoes (and baked pumpkin and greens as well). The possibilities of spuds are endless. But you do need good ones – otherwise you're condemned to grainy mash. Potatoes have only slightly more calories than apples. For centuries potatoes were the main winter source of vitamin C, with roughly the same amount of iron per spud as in an egg. They're also high in roughage and potassium. Potatoes are good for you.

### *Harvesting potatoes*

Harvest potatoes when all the potato vegetation has died down. Put them in hessian bags or wooden boxes covered in newspaper straight away. Potatoes turn green very fast when first dug and exposed to sunlight, and green potatoes are poisonous.

*Fresh eating* All year with planning, except in very hot areas. Crops can be heavily mulched where the ground freezes, or grown in warm piles of tyres.

*Storage time* About three months, away from light and moisture in the cool of the year.

*Food value* 335 kj per 100 g – about the same as apples. High in vitamin C, potassium, some niacine, thiamine, protein and phosphorus.

### *Leaving potatoes in the ground*

I never store potatoes – not above-ground anyway. Potatoes can be left in the ground till you need them. If they start to grow again you'll just have a new crop of spuds. Potatoes won't start to grow anyway for at least six weeks after the tops die back, and often not till the next season.

Potatoes will survive heavy frosts above them, but they won't tolerate frozen ground. If your ground freezes during winter, dig them up before it does, or cover the ground thickly with mulch or sand for insulation.

### *Potato bandicooting*

We have a wild patch of potatoes – it keeps growing, as we never entirely harvest the crop. I just wriggle my hand down and pull out what we need. Any weeds in that part of the garden, old corn stalks, prunings, etc. are tossed onto the potatoes – the only mulch and feeding they get. They've been feeding us for ten years.

Note that this doesn't work in an area where lots of people are growing potatoes and aphids may spread disease from one crop to another. In that case you need to buy in fresh seed potatoes every year and plant them in a different part of the garden.

### *Potatoes for storage*

Potatoes for storage should be harvested when the tops wither. The skins are tougher and will stay firm longer. Always bag your potatoes as soon as you bring them above ground – they are most prone to 'greening' when just dug.

Store them in a dark, airy place where they won't sweat. A vegetable rack is best. Damp potatoes rot. Never store them in plastic bags. Don't store potatoes near apples or citrus either – most fruit releases ethylene which promotes ripening, causing your potatoes to sprout prematurely and turn soft.

Clean your potato storage area after every crop – that way any spores from past rotting won't affect the next lot.

### *How to cook a potato*

#### *Boiling*

Scrub your potatoes – don't peel them. The peel will rub off when they are cooked and keeping it on helps keep the potato firm. New potatoes should be plunged into boiling water. For old potatoes, just cover with cold water and bring to the boil VERY slowly. Add a little lemon juice or peel to old potatoes to keep them white.

When they are almost done (about fifteen minutes of boiling) drain off the water and put the lid on. This way the potatoes finish cooking in steam, not water and won't explode.

#### *Steaming*

I use a bamboo steamer. Again, leave the potatoes whole or they'll turn grainy. Steamed potatoes take about half an hour to cook, but have a slightly better flavour than boiled ones.

#### *Baking*

Preheat the oven to about 250°C. Scrub the potatoes, don't peel them. Pierce them a couple of times with a fork to let the steam escape so they don't explode. They'll take an hour to an hour and a half to cook. Hold them in a tea towel and peel and dress while still warm.

*Cooking new potatoes*
Cover your potatoes with cold water, bring them very slowly to the boil, turn down the heat and simmer till they are *nearly* cooked. Now put a lid covered with two teatowels over the saucepan and let them finish cooking in their own heat. This method gives firm new potatoes, without ragged split skins and fuzzy overcooked patches at the bottom.

*Potatoes in the microwave*
Place your unpeeled, unsliced, pierced potatoes in a covered dish with a little water. They'll take about ten minutes, depending on their size. Take them out before they are fully cooked and let the heat in the dish finish the cooking.

*POTATO FLOUR*
Slice, dry and grind potatoes for potato flour. Potato flour used to be one of the emergency foods in colonial Australia – whenever the flour went weevily, or drowned in the creek on the way from town, you turned to potato flour – or even just mashed potatoes added to your bread dough. Use one part potato flour to three parts wheat flour in bread, cakes, etc. Use dried potato for thickening. Make potato cakes from mashed or grated raw potato, sautéed or deep fried, with cheese, ham, other vegetables, or fish – potato is an excellent base for almost anything. Use mashed potato instead of pastry to make a pie base. Use a quarter mashed potato instead of flour in cake recipes.

*CHIPS*
Dry potatoes well, and plunge them in hot oil – not too many or the oil will cool and they'll be greasy. When they are just starting to brown take them out, heat the oil again, then plunge the chips in a second time till brown.

### *POTATO SALAD*

Potato salads suffer from being popular. Most are awful. Potato salads are the white dab on the plate next to the fried chicken or singed steak, tasting of vinegar and possessing a texture like frayed wool.

You can taste the potato in a good potato salad – as well as the other ingredients. In fact this is the test of a good potato salad: it should be a gentle marrying of flavours and textures, not invasion and domination. Like bread, potatoes are subtle enough to combine with an enormous number of other flavours and textures – but unless you can still tell there's potato there, the exercise is pointless. And like the countless sorts of bread, every culture that grows potatoes has its own potato salads.

Never try to make a potato salad with grainy or collapsing potatoes. Mash them or make soup instead. It is the dressing that contains most of the calories in potato salad – and most commercial potato salads have a lot of dressing. If you use firm, flavoursome, home-grown potatoes you won't need so much dressing.

### *CLASSIC POTATO SALAD*

This is simply diced or sliced potatoes, dressed – preferably while still warm – with either mayonnaise (garlic mayonnaise or aïoli is even better) or with salad cream. Optional extras include diced fried bacon or ham, chopped apple, walnuts, chopped parsley, coriander, mustard or watercress.

If you find mayonnaise makes the salad too thick for your liking, thin it with a little milk or (sour) cream. This will make the texture more like 'conventional' potato salad. I prefer my dressing undiluted.

### *VAGUELY ASIAN POTATO SALAD*

1 kilo sliced cooked potatoes
1 teaspoon ground cardamom
1 teaspoon cumin
1 teaspoon lemon juice
1 cup natural yogurt
chopped coriander

Heat all ingredients except the potatoes; pour over the potatoes and leave till cool. Serve chilled.

*POTATOES WITH PEANUT SAUCE*

1 kilo sliced cooked potatoes

Dressing:

$^1/_2$ a cup of peanut butter
1 tablespoon soy sauce
2 chopped chillies (can be omitted)
5 tablespoons tomato purée
4 tablespoons oil
$^1/_2$ a cup of lemon juice
brown sugar to taste

Mix the dressing well, pour over the potatoes. If it is too thick a little more tomato purée or water can be added – you should be able to scoop it easily with a spoon.

Serve hot or cold.

*STUFFED POTATO SALAD*

Take a warm, large baked potato. Cut the top off carefully. Gently hollow it out with a teaspoon – you want the innards in chunks, not as a mash. Add any of the following to the potato pieces:
finely chopped celery
chopped artichoke hearts
chopped chives
chopped parsley
a very little chervil
chopped fried bacon
chopped red capsicum (only if you are going to eat it straight away)
pickled cucumber

Dress with mayonnaise or vinaigrette, yoghurt or tahini dressing (I prefer mayonnaise). Stuff it *gently* back into the potato. Replace the lid at an angle, so you can see the stuffing oozing out.

These are best served by themselves, and not with other salads or mixed meats.

### *POTATO CAKES*

For every cup of grated potato add 1 dessertspoon chopped parsley, 2 chopped cloves of garlic, 1 dessertspoon chopped onion, 1 egg, and 1 tablespoon plain flour. Mix well. Drop spoonfuls in a hot pan with plenty of olive oil or butter. Cook till brown on one side, then turn.

If the cake sticks, the pan wasn't hot enough, or clean enough. If the potatoes are very liquid you may need to add a little more flour.

### *GRATIN DAUPHINOISE*

Slice potatoes thinly – use firm waxy ones if possible – certainly not old ones in spring that will be grainy as they are beginning to get ready to sprout.

Lay them in a dish with a little chopped onion if you like, or chopped garlic. Cover with cream or sour cream or a mixture of either with stock. Place in a slow oven and bake.

The top will become crusty and brown and delicious, the inside will be rich and creamy as the liquid evaporates and is taken up by the spuds. This dish is good by itself, not as an accompaniment to anything, except perhaps a green salad.

### *DRIED POTATO*

Grate the potato (peeled or not, according to preference) and spread as thinly as possible on alfoil in the sun. Should dry in a day or two.

### *POTATO CHEESES*

Take 2 kg mashed potatoes, very finely mashed. Add half a litre of sour milk or cream, and beat well. Leave in a china dish covered with a tea towel in a cool place (not the fridge) for four days. Knead the mixture well, then place small rounds in muslin or cloth to drain for two days. Rub the cheeses over with butter. They should mature for at least three weeks and will keep well for years.

### *POTATO BREAD*

This is lighter and stores better than ordinary bread.

4 cups plain flour – wholemeal or white

1 cup potato flour or dry mashed potato (pumpkin flour can also be used)
1 teaspoon dried yeast
water

Place the yeast in the warm water with a little flour. Leave till it bubbles. Now combine the flours, add the yeast, and enough water to make it bind. Knead for at least 20 minutes. Leave to rise in a warm place – I cover it with a teatowel and put it near the stove or on the window sill. Punch it down, and let it rise again to double its bulk. Bake in a hot oven till the top is brown and springs back when you press it. The sides of the loaf will have shrunk back from the sides of the tin.

# *pumpkins*

*This takes up a great deal of ground, with its large thick creeping stalks, furnished with large claspers its leaves are large and rough, like those of melons. The flowers are large, like a yellow lily in colour. The fruit is large, having large white flattish oval seeds. It is grown on dunghills.*

NICHOLAS CULPEPPER

***If you can grow*** pumpkins ***you can grow*** watermelons ***or*** rock melons . . . ***and*** cucumbers ***too (though as they're smaller they need more weed control) or*** perennial squash.

### *ROOTS*

Cinderella rode in a pumpkin – which was a waste of a good pumpkin (but maybe the good fairy had pumpkin pie next evening as a celebratory dinner). Pumpkins are native to North America and were not introduced to Europe till the 16th century – so Cinderella must be relatively modern.

Pumpkins used to be the old colonial standby – even if nothing else grew: the cockies in the corn, the wallabies in the orchard, the drought destroying the lettuce – you'd still have pumpkins. Pumpkin flour was used in bread to partially replace wheat flour – and most of us know all about pumpkin scones. In colonial days, all you had to do to grow your pumpkins was to find a creek flat, wait for a spring flood, then plant the seeds in the silt. Off you went shearing – to come back in autumn to pick your pumpkin crop.

## *MEDICINAL PUMPKINS*

An old cure for tapeworms was squeezing out the gel from unripe pumpkins and eating that before bedtime – the contents of three or four seeds was an adult dose. I haven't tried it, nor do I intend to. I gather the side effects can be spectacular – and you'll need a dunny handy the next day. Eating whole pumpkin seeds has also been claimed to help get rid of tapeworm.

Like all yellow/orange foods rich in beta carotene, a diet high in pumpkin may help ward off a range of cancers, heart disease, strokes and cataracts, and generally help raise the body's immunity to disease.

## *SOME PUMPKIN VARIETIES*

### *Bush pumpkins*

These don't spread. You can grow them neatly in the garden or in a pot, including inside in winter. The pumpkins are usually small – one meal's worth – and mature very quickly.

*Butterbush* A small fruited butternut on a small vine. Stores well.

*Bush Table Queen* This gives dark green acorn shaped fruit with thick dry flesh.

*Golden Nugget* This is one of the most popular bush pumpkins – round gold fruit on a non-running bush. Can be eaten quite small (with luck you'll even have them for Christmas even in cool areas) or left to mature. They store remarkably well.

### *Medium sized vines*

Butternut, Hercules Butternut, Butternut Waltham: all the familiar supermarket butternuts, but they'll taste better if they're from your garden.

### *Large vines*

*Queensland Blue* Old-fashioned hard grey, good keeper.

*Windsor Black* Dark green skin, good flavour, early maturing.

*Turk's Turban* Bright orange, hard skinned fruit to 25 cm across, with a 'Turk's hat' on top. Very good keeper.

*Jarrahdale* One of the best flavours and textures, with grey skin and deep orange flesh – a wonderful baking pumpkin.

### *Huge pumpkins*

These are often watery and/or stringy and not very good: cattle pumpkins. But they are great to boast about, or to use to replace the kitchen table.

*Big Max* Huge fruit, to two metres.

*Prizewinner* Huge, golden fruit up to 90 kg: a hybrid variety.

### *Perennial Squash/ Chilacayote melons*

These die down in the frost, though in mild winters here, with frosts of no more than minus 5°C, ours have survived. The vines climb seven metres up the avocado trees, down to the flat then up a wattle tree – with massive, great round melons hanging all over it, ready to fall and give you concussion if you're walking underneath.

The 'melons' can be cooked like squash, baked like pumpkin or eaten raw in fruit salad – well sweetened, as they are pretty flavourless. A good 'bulking' food. With a vine of chilacayote melons you'll never starve.

A word of warning: you need an axe to cut through them – but they last for years.

## *CULTIVATION*

### *Why you should grow your own*

Don't eat the skin of commercial pumpkins in case they have been treated with fungicides.

### *Essential information*

Pumpkins are a frost tender annual.

Feed them well and don't let the vine take over your garden. That's probably all you need to say about pumpkins – they grow themselves, though nowadays you are more likely to see them sprouting from compost heaps than dungheaps.

I plant our pumpkins on top of shovels full of compost or well rotted manure – two seeds per heap, then pull out the weakest. Feed young vines well – I use decomposed hen manure. Well fed and watered pumpkins will outgrow weeds and even ramble through grass and over blackberries and lantana – but they *must* be well fed. Young plants however must be kept mulched or weeded. Pumpkins do best in humus rich soil.

It's almost impossible to overfeed pumpkins (I've seen one grow over a metre a day in hot weather). Pile on the manure, as Culpepper advises, and give plenty of water. You can also feed with hen manure every week – start with a dessertspoon every week and build up to two cups a week as it grows. Keep feeding as long as the vine keeps flowering.

Don't plant your pumpkins in the garden bed – they'll spread and crowd out the lettuces and beans. Train them up a trellis instead, or plant them at the edge of the garden and train them outwards.

If you want a giant pumpkin for the show, insert a little strand of cotton wool in the base of the stalk, and leave one end in a saucer of nine parts water and one part urine.

### *Keeping pumpkin seed*

The riper the melon or pumpkin the more likely that the seed will germinate. You can plant the seed from a shop-bought melon or pumpkin. Unfortunately most ripe melons and pumpkins come mid or late season (unless they have been kept fromthe season before). The early ones are rarely ripe enough, so that when you do get the seed it is too late to plant it. Dry it for next year. Melon and pumpkin seed should be hard shelled when they are ripe, unless they are Pepita or Triple Treat pumpkins with hull-less seeds.

Choose the best pumpkin in your garden for pumpkin seed. Wait till the stem is brittle and dry before you pick it. Let it stand for a few weeks before you take out the seed, so it matures completely.

Pumpkins come true to type unless there is another variety nearby – and then you can get some interesting variations. Unfortunately there is a good chance there may be flowering pumpkins nearby – if only escapees from someone's compost heap. Unless you are saving a rare variety however, you may not mind this. I rather enjoy waiting to see what pumpkins the vines produce each year – though I've carefully covered flowers on precious varieties with bags, and hand-pollinated the female flowers (the ones with bulges at the bottom) with pollen from the males to make sure they breed true.

Pumpkin seeds last about 5 to 10 years. Store them in an old envelope in a dry spot – and make sure rats and mice can't get to them.

### *When to sow*

For those who lack a flood prone creek flat, sow pumpkin seeds as follows:

*Tropical areas* All year round, but you may have problems in humid months.

*Subtropical areas* July to February.

*Temperate areas* September to December. You may get away with a small crop of the tiny pumpkins in January/February if the weather remains hot.

*Cool areas* October to December.

### *Germination and yield*

*Germination temperatures* 10-32°C, but does best if the temperature is over 18°C.

*Seedlings emerge* 6 to 10 days.

*Time until your first pumpkin* 14 to 16 weeks, depending on warmth and variety, but most vines will keep producing for months after the first pumpkin is ready.

*Number of vines needed for a family of four* Who knows? This will depend on where you live (longer growing seasons mean more pumpkins), on how big the pumpkins are and how much you eat. Most backyard growers probably plant two bush pumpkins for an early crop, and two to four vines for big pumpkins – but you may find the bush ones are enough, or you may like 10 vines and the security of knowing that no matter what else happens in the world, with the harvest from ten pumpkin vines, you'll never starve.

### *Pumpkins in autumn*

If you are afraid your pumpkins won't mature in cool seasons, nip off the later flowers so all the strength goes into maturing the oldest fruit.

Hang vines up in the shed at the end of autumn, roots, soil and all – the pumpkins (or melons) will continue to ripen. Eat small pumpkins the way you would zucchini – either immature ones or ones you don't need as whoppers. Pumpkin flowers can also be eaten: stuff them or fry them. Nip off the ends of pumpkin vines in late summer to speed up the maturing pumpkins.

Pick melons and pumpkins when the stalks wither.

### *Seven ways to grow a pumpkin*

Pumpkins are messy creatures. Unless you grow the bush variety they sprawl all over the place. But if you like the old-fashioned ramblers – Queensland Blue, Butternut, or Paw Paw pumpkins – the following might help keep your pumpkins from strangling the tomatoes overnight.

#### *Pumpkins on the lawn*

You don't need to use the front lawn for this – any bit of waste space at the back will do.

Take a spadeful of compost. If you don't have compost, buy some good potting mix instead. Lay down a bit of newspaper, about three pages thick. Lay your compost on top. Plant a pumpkin seedling. Water well.

By the time the pumpkin sticks its roots into the soil under the paper it will be big and strong and able to outgrow the grass. Keep the grass well mown while you can – after a while though it will be smothered in pumpkin leaves. I've found pumpkins in grass mature slightly faster than those grown in garden beds – the grass perhaps helps insulate the vines.

#### *Pumpkins in weeds*

Remember that pile of rotting weeds down the back? Make a small depression at the top, add a spadeful of compost or soil, plant a pumpkin seedling. This is the fastest way I know to get a crop of pumpkins. The heat from the rotting weeds speeds up the vine – and the extra watering you give the pumpkin speeds up decomposition. This means that the nutrients from the rotting weeds are available to give you a giant crop.

*Pumpkins in tyres*
Scavenge two old tyres from the local garage. Pile them on top of each other. Fill with grass clippings, then compost or soil and then a seedling as above. Black absorbs warmth and the vine will surge ahead.

In frosty areas try a pile three to six tyres high. This will need a stake down the middle to stop them falling over. Fill with rocks or any old material at the bottom to save on grass clippings or soil. The vine will trail down the tyres and the extra height and heat will help protect the vine from early frosts.

*Pumpkins in alfoil*
This gives your vine an early start in cool areas. Stretch a metre of alfoil over some grass. Cut a small hole and plant your seedling. Water very well and preferably give liquid fertiliser every three days till it's growing well and will outcompete the now rotting grass under the alfoil. Place a plastic bottle with the bottom cut out over the seedling at night to protect it against late frosts.

Don't try this in hot areas – the seedling will burn.

*Pumpkins in weed mat*
Try the same technique with weed mat. Again, the black mat will absorb heat. You don't need to remove the grass first. I just lay down weed mat on any spare lawn or weedy garden, cut a hole and plant.

*Pumpkins on a sheet of newspaper*
Lay the newspaper on the grass, place a shovel full of compost on top. Then stick in the seeds. Water well and feed when young.

*Vertical pumpkins*
Grow your pumpkins up a trellis. They'll mature faster up in the air, be less prone to mildew, and you can count the crop every day as you pass.

### *COMPANION PLANTING WITH PUMPKINS*

Let pumpkin vines wander up trees and trellises so the leaves aren't splashed with mildew spores from the ground. The air circulation will also be better. I find avocado trees an excellent support for pumpkins, but wattles, apples, grevilleas and reinforcing mesh do as well.

## *GROWING PAINS*

### *Mildews*

Prune off affected leaves as soon as they appear. Limit overhead watering. Water in the morning so the leaves don't stay wet overnight. Stake the vine to let air circulate round the leaves. Grow on top of mulch to avoid soil contact.

Grow pumpkins on weed mat, use a newspaper mulch or grow the vines in well-mown grass instead of in a humid vegetable garden where the air can't move and is full of moisture evaporating from the vegies. Bordeaux spray can be used in cool weather, but make sure it doesn't touch any flowers or new leaves. Powdery mildew can also be treated with Condy's crystals dissolved in water. Actively growing pumpkins in well-fed soil are more resistant to mildew.

### *Aphids*

Aphids cause twisted leaves, but pumpkins usually grow so strongly these don't matter. Squash them between your fingers on new shoots.

### *Thrips*

Keep pumpkins growing strongly and thrips (small insects in the flowers) won't be a problem.

## *FROM THE GARDEN TO THE TABLE*

### *Harvest*

Bush pumpkins like Golden Nuggets can bear 4-10 fruit. Large vines may produce between 3 and 25 fruit – a few in cool climates, many more in hot areas with well-fed plants.

Pumpkins are ripe when the stalk is dry next to the fruit, or breaks off. 'Ripe' pumpkins have tougher skins, store better and

are sweeter as well. But a pumpkin can be picked at any time – it just won't be as sweet. Serve it with sauce, butter, etc. instead.
*Fresh eating period* About the frost free period minus 100 days, but long keepers may survive for six months, so it is possible to have fresh pumpkin all year. Grow Butternuts or Early Butter pumpkins as well as keepers like Jarrahdale and Queensland Blue
*Storage time* Eight months for long keepers 'cured' on the roof or in a dry spot in the sun for two weeks after picking. Don't pick for storage till the stalk withers. Use unmatured pumpkins like baby squash – steamed or baked with butter and garlic.

A word of warning: *Never* use pumpkin that has gone off, you may get food poisoning. I find that pumpkin pie and pumpkin soup can go off faster than any other other pie or soup I know. Keep them cool, and get rid of them if you have the slightest doubt about their soundness.
*Food value* 130 kj per 100 g. High vitamin A, some vitamin C, potassium, iron and calcium.

### *Storing pumpkins*

You can't beat a hot tin roof. The heat 'cures' the pumpkins by slightly baking them – the skins harden and any fungi spores are killed. If you don't have a dunny or a garden shed (the classic places to cure a pumpkin) place them on concrete or paving for a few days instead, turning them every day. Take them in when it rains though, and before frosts.

Make sure you always store your pumpkins *on their sides*. Otherwise moisture will condense on the top or bottom, and the pumpkin will start rotting.

Then enjoy a good eight months of pumpkin eating.

### *How to peel a pumpkin*

If you doubt your wrist power, don't bother – cook it with the skin on, then take it off later, or eat it. Some skins are delicious and good roughage – others are sharp, tough and horrible. Otherwise bung the pumpkin in a very hot oven for a few minutes to soften the skin, cool and peel.

The best way to cut a pumpkin like a Queensland Blue or Jarrahdale is to put it on the bench, stick a knife in the centre –

like stabbing an enemy – then press downwards rather than cut, so the knife slides though one of the grooves in the pumpkin. It is more complicated to write about it than to do it.

### *Coping with surplus pumpkins*

It's easy to get a 'pumpkin emergency' when you've cut a chunk from a pumpkin and don't know what to do with the rest, or one has started to go off and you want to use the sound bit.

Add one-third mashed pumpkin instead of flour to bread and cakes to make them light and moist. Do the same with pikelets, then sprinkle them with sugar or spread them with honey – wonderful. Mashed pumpkin can be frozen. Stuff whole pumpkins and bake. Make pumpkin instead of potato salad. Use pumpkin instead of potato in potato or fish cakes. Try baked pumpkin with a sauce of cream and french mustard boiled for three minutes.

#### *PUMPKIN FLOUR*

This can be made the same way as sweet potato flour, but omit the lemon juice. Pumpkin flour is good added to cakes – one cup of pumpkin flour to four cups of ordinary flour.

#### *MOCK GINGER*

This is an old colonial standby.

Chop your pumpkin into neat slices, sprinkle with salt and leave overnight. Pour off the juice. Add a syrup of two cups of sugar to one cup of water and a dessertspoon of grated or powdered ginger. Boil for an hour, pour over the pumpkin, leave till cold. Pour off the syrup and repeat at least six times. The pumpkin should look as though it is starting to candy and change colour with the repeated applications of boiling syrup. Put the lot in the oven till the pumpkin is cooked. The outside will still be crunchy due to its crystallising but the inside will be soft. Place in clean jars while hot with a shaving of lemon zest. Seal. Don't use for at least three months. This keeps for years.

#### *BAKED PUMPKIN*

This is of course exquisite with roast lamb or beef – the top is caramelised and the bottom absorbs some of the meat juices. But it's also good fried on both sides till brown in a teflon frypan (no fat, few calories) then baked till tender.

*PUMPKIN 'OVENS'*

In colonial days, if you lacked a pot, a stew was often put in a hollowed-out pumpkin then put beside the fire or buried in hot ashes to cook slowly. You can also use this method in the oven. The pumpkin 'reseals' itself and the effect is a bit like a pressure cooker, or a very well-sealed casserole. The result is extremely good, as none of the flavour can escape.

Cut the top off your pumpkin – a large one for a family, small for individual serves. Fill with your favourite casserole – or even stock, for a good soup. Replace the lid exactly as it was before. Cook *slowly*, and eat hot.

*PUMPKIN SOUP*

Mash two cups of cooked pumpkin into four cups of chicken stock, or vegetable stock enriched with tomato purée. I like to add an onion and six cloves of garlic sautéed in a little butter too.

Blend the whole lot. Add cream if you feel like it and perhaps a sprinkle of nutmeg, cinnamon, parsley or even finely grated orange zest.

*BAKED CHOKO AND PUMPKIN*

This is an old Michael Boddy recipe – a weird combination but it works.

Layer thin slices of alternating pumpkin and choko in an oven dish and dot with butter (or just make sure the pan is well oiled). Bake slowly for two hours. Incredibly sweet and good.

*PUMPKIN CURRY*

Pumpkin is both sweet and meat in a curry – and good.

1 teaspoonful of cumin, coriander, turmeric, and garam masala
2 cups peeled chopped tomatoes, or 1 can tomatoes
2 cups chopped pumpkin (hoose a firm, finely grained one.)
2 onions, chopped
12 cloves of garlic, chopped
3 tablespoons olive oil

chilli to taste (I use two chopped red chillies for a medium hot curry.)

Cook the onions and garlic slowly in the oil till soft, add the spices and stir well for a few minutes. Don't let them burn. Add the other ingredients and simmer till the pumpkin is cooked.

For the best flavour leave the curry in the fridge overnight and reheat it the next day.

*BLOODY GOOD PUMPKIN SCONES*

1 tablespoon honey
1 teaspoon grated orange zest
2 tablespoons butter
1 cup mashed pumpkin – as orange and sweet as you can get it
1 well beaten egg
$^{1}/_{2}$ a cup of milk
2 cups self-raising flour

Mix the orange zest with the flour, work the butter and honey in with your fingers. Add the milk and egg and pumpkin – work as little as you can at this stage. Now cut into thin rounds – about as thick as the width of your thumb. Brush with milk or beaten egg, bake in a hot oven for 10 – 15 minutes.

These scones should be eaten fresh. If there are any left over, toast them for breakfast (toasted breakfast scones were a feature of staying with my Grandmother) or cut them into slices and bake in the oven till crisp and crush for very superior 'breadcrumbs'.

*PUMPKIN SEEDS*

These can be delicious. Try to get them before they are fully matured, from unripe pumpkins. They'll be more tender.

Wash them well and scrub off any bits of fibre. Toss them in an oiled pan with a little garlic or chilli, or salt them later. Fry till brown, turn and brown again. Eat hot or cold.

As pumpkin seeds get older, the outside skin gets too hard to eat. You then need to crack it and remove the centre. You can also buy a 'hull-less' pumpkin like Triple Treat, where the seeds don't develop hard shells. There are stringy pumpkins and poor keepers – and the seeds aren't really worth it when you can eat the seeds of other pumpkins young.

*PUMPKIN FLOWERS*

Pick the male ones (those that don't have a bulbous bit at the stem end). Fry them in butter and sprinkle with icing sugar, or stuff with fried rice and cook in chicken stock or tomato purée or lemon juice. Or dip them in sweet or plain batter and eat with garlic mayonnaise or lemon juice and icing sugar.

*PUMPKIN TENDRILS*

These are edible too and can be good (avoid them when bitter). Snip them off and stir fry them quickly till they turn bright instead of dull green. Good and crunchy.

# *tomatoes*

*In Spain and those hot regions they eat the Apples prepared and boiled with pepper, salt and oyle, buyt they yled very little nourishment to the body, and the same naught and corupt.*
GERARD, *The Herball or Historie of Plants*, 1597

***If you can grow a*** tomato ***you can also grow*** eggplant (aubergine), chillies, rosellas, capsicum ***and*** okra

### *ROOTS*

Tomatoes were originally a South American weed. The word tomato comes from the ancient Mexican word for tomato: *tomatl*. Christopher Columbus took them to Europe where they were received with suspicion as being poisonous, suitable only to grow as an ornamental *pomo dei mori* (apple of the Moors or apple of death, anglicised to Golden Apples), and later as *Pomme d'amour* – 'love apples' or aphrodisiacs.

The sweet varieties we know today are fairly recent – most early tomato recipes added sugar or honey.

### *TOMATOES AND HEALTH*

Tomatoes are high in vitamin C and contain lycopene, an antioxidant.

Tomatoes can be too acid for anyone who suffers from heartburn. Yellow tomato varieties are often less acidic. Tomatoes can also trigger migraines in a small number of people. A tomato-rich diet has been linked to lower levels of pancreatic cancer, lung cancer and cervical cancers (as well as precancerous CIN, cervical intraepithelial neoplasia) and other forms of cancer.

Women with high levels of lycopenes (found mostly in tomatoes and watermelon) are five times less likely to develop CIN according to studies at the University of Illinois. One study of lung cancer victims indicated that those with a diet high in oranges and tomatoes in particular had higher survival rates.

Some five per cent of arthritis sufferers believe that avoiding tomatoes, as well as other solanums, relieves their symptoms.

## *TOMATO VARIETIES*

This is a matter of argument between gardeners. Most tomato growers have their favourite variety that they feel is sweeter and has a fuller flavour. To some extent which tomato you like depends on what you will use it for: crinkly juicy ones don't slice well for sandwiches, perfect slicing tomatoes don't have the 'meat' that good cooking tomatoes do.

There are hundreds of tomato varieties – eat your way through them. This year we are growing climbing yellow ones (prolific and frost hardy), egg shaped Roma (sweet), Tiny Tim that come up anyway from the ones I planted ten years ago and a couple of large ones. I usually plant an early-bearing variety in spring and a late-bearing variety in December.

Others worth trying are yellow climbing tomato (a fairly late but prolific bearer, though the fruit is slightly bland), Rouge de Marmande that crops even in cool areas, Tiny Tim or cherry tomatoes – and there are dozens of others.

I planted a 'Siberian' tomato this year, said to germinate at 4°C. The seedlings appeared after every other variety was reaching for the sky – and now, come December, they're still only finger high. Maybe they only work in Siberia – or maybe the seed was infected with a virus. (I'm taking them to the dump in a plastic bag tomorrow.)

If you are looking for cold climate tomatoes, look for ones with large leaves and pronounced crinkles so they can absorb the maximum amount of sunlight.

Digger's Club Seeds conduct 'tomato tasting' tests. They reckon 'Tommy Toe' (a large 'cherry' type) has the best flavour. Their Mortgage lifter tomato gave the most fruit (14.494 kilos) followed by Green Zebra and the hybrid Apollo. They also sell a drying tomato, striped tomatoes, an enormous range of green and yellow tomatoes, cooking tomatoes – in fact, you'll find a tomato to suit any taste or desire. Strongly recommended for all tomato lovers.

Keep a lookout for climbing tomatoes. They will ramble up a trellis – and you get an enormous amount of fruit from a very small space. They trail down tubs beautifully too.

## *CULTIVATION*

### *Why you should grow your own*

Tomatoes will be sprayed and probably fumigated for fruit fly. Fumigants include: EDB (ethylene dibromide) and methyl bromide. The US Food and Drug Administration permits less than 10 micro grams per gram of residue after fumigation with an inorganic bromide. (Heat and chilling are pollutant free alternatives to fruit fly fumigation.) EDB is extremely carcinogenic in animal tests and there are plans to phase it out in Australia. Methyl bromide's use is restricted – it is possibly carcinogenic and mutagenic. It is odourless and tasteless.

### *Essential information*

Tomatoes are a short-lived perennial, usually grown as an annual in temperate to cold areas and in disease-prone hot areas. This means, basically, that most tomatoes rarely last longer than one season.

Plant tomatoes when the soil is warm and again a few months later. Start tomatoes indoors in cold weather and transplant when the soil reaches 20°C. I also plant a cherry tomato in late summer. These are more frost hardy than most tomatoes and will crop in a sheltered space through most of winter. The tiny winter tomatoes aren't very sweet – but they do add colour to a salad.

You can sow seeds directly where they are to grow if you wish, but most people raise theirs indoors or cover the seedling pot with plastic first to get earlier tomatoes.

*Don't* bother trying to grow tomatoes too early (see temperatures above). Tomatoes that are started in cold soil sulk and actually bear later and often less than those sown at the optimum time.

Pick tomatoes as soon a they are ripe, or even starting to colour in fruit fly prone areas and pick up all fallen ones.

### *Saving tomato seed*

Choose ripe, red tomatoes, the best you can find – preferably from the lower branches, but this isn't essential. Then leave them on the window sill to ripen further. When they are too squashy to tempt you to eat them, let them ferment in a jar of water (don't stir – just let them foam and bubble), then separate the seeds and dry them. The fermentation kills a range of seed borne diseases.

If you leave the seeds fermenting too long, they'll germinate almost as soon as you take them out. Only leave them for two to three days, then dry them on newspaper.

Seedling tomatoes often spring up from last year's tomato bed. Cherish the best of them, and you'll gradually select a tomato variety perfectly suited to your garden.

Seeds last between three and six years.

### *When to sow*

*Tropical areas* All year round.

*Subtropical areas* All year round – protect from the odd frost.

*Temperate areas* When the soil is warm enough to sit on comfortably (traditionally bare bummed but that isn't essential) – usually August to December.

*Cool areas* August/September indoors, transplant outdoors in October or when soil temperature reaches 20°C. Can be planted till early December or even January for tiny cherry tomatoes.

### *Germination and yield*

*Germination temperatures* 18-26°C. Start seeds indoors and transplant when soil temperature is at least 20°C.

*Fruit set* Between 20-28°C.

*Seedlings emerge* 10 to 14 days.

*Time to your first tomato* About 10 to 20 weeks, depending on climate and variety. Cherry tomatoes are much earlier and crop later into the cool of the year. Tomatoes will crop till the next frost or till they die of wilt or other diseases – at least three months, hopefully much longer, even years. In temperate areas you may find your grafted tomatoes bear again next summer.

*Number of plants needed for a family of four* 12 to 24 for fresh eating and a reasonable amount of tomato sauce and dried tomatoes.

*Yield* Probably about 5 kg per plant, but good plants will yield from 10 to 60 kg per plant.

*Successions* Young tomatoes are more disease resistant so plant tomatoes every two or three months or take cuttings of the last lot and plant them as far away as practicable from the others or let old branches root – see below.

### *Growing tomatoes*

#### *Mulching*

Tomatoes form roots up their stems and stalk if they are mulched. The more roots, the better they grow – so mulch right up to the stem if you can. I don't bother to stake my tomatoes initially – the branches that sprawl on the ground take root, then I stake them up and have another tomato plant.

#### *Pruning*

Don't bother to prune tomatoes – they ripen in response to heat, not sunlight. Pruning is just one more task that gardeners have burdened themselves with. If you are a pruning fanatic prune the tomatoes to two stems, or laterals. The lateral below the first flower truss is usually the most vigorous – but as I said, why bother?

#### *Staking tomatoes*

Staked tomatoes look neat. Unstaked ones fall over and the branches sprawl all over the place, but sprawling tomato branches form roots on the bottom so the tomato vine is much more vigorous. A good idea, as long as you don't mind wading through a couple of acres of plant while you look for ripe tomatoes.

If you are going to stake your tomatoes (through innate tidiness or because your gardening fanatic father who always stakes his is coming to visit and you don't want to argue about tomato growing methods), use old stockings or bits of cloth, rather than string which can cut into the soft branches. Don't tie too tightly as you can cut off circulation as the branches grow bigger. Just loop the stocking round the branch very loosely, then loop it again around the stake. This gives leeway in windy weather so branches are less likely to snap if pulled away from the stake.

*Watering tomatoes*

Try to avoid overhead watering – it can splash disease spores up onto the leaves and increase humidity so fruit splits and fungal and mildew problems increase. Slip the hose under the mulch if possible, or use trickle irrigation. If you must overhead water, do it in the evening (contrary to most advice): morning watering means they'll be wet in the heat of the day – which most disease spores love.

Another solution is to plant the tomatoes on slightly raised rows, then make furrows between the rows and water the furrows.

*Feeding tomatoes*

It is almost impossible to overfeed tomatoes – that's why they spring up in badly treated sewerage and chook yards among almost pure manure. We picked 40 kilos from one bush once that sprang up at the end of the hen house in almost pure hen droppings – then we gave up counting. Don't starve the poor things or they'll be stingy producers.

The more you feed tomatoes, the more you'll get. If you don't feed them – even if your soil is naturally fertile – you probably won't get a decent crop.

Tomatoes need ample potash and phosphorus as well as nitrogen. They thrive on hen manure and will tolerate higher doses of fresh hen manure than most other plants, though this might produce masses of leaves and few fruit.

Phosphorus deficiency is indicated by purple tinged leaves. Scatter on rock phosphate, mulch with compost or feed with hen manure or another phosphorus and potash rich fertiliser. A green manure crop of barley will make phosphorus more available to tomatoes.

Avoid too much nitrogen when the plant is young or you may get a massive bush with few tomatoes. There are three excellent ways of providing tomatoes with the phosphorus they need without giving them too much nitrogen:

- Plant the tomatoes in a trench filled with comfrey or compost or use compost or comfrey mulch.
- Use a green manure fertiliser once a week.
- Grow a green manure barley crop and slash it before planting out the tomatoes.

Feed your tomatoes with a high-nitrogen fertiliser when the plant begins to flower as its nitrogen needs rise then. Fruiting tomatoes are very hungry plants. A weekly dose of dolomite, quick-fix or soluble fertiliser is excellent, though if you have fed your tomatoes with compost or a good quality mulch the nutrients will be readily available by the time the tomato begins to flower and no other feeding should be necessary, as long as you keep renewing the mulch.

Well-fed tomatoes crop for a much longer period than those forced with too much nitrogen. Nitrogen starved tomatoes have pale green leaves tinged with purple.

If your tomato flowers drop off before setting fruit your soil may be too acid. Add lime, dolomite or – even better – wood ash.

Blotchy tomatoes, with hard yellow patches on ripe or near-ripe tomatoes, are suffering from potash or phosphorus deficiency. Try a foliar spray made from potash and phosphorus rich materials like seaweed, hen manure, comfrey and urine.

Blossom end rot, which shows as a dark patch on the plant, is due to irregular watering or lack of calcium. Mulch well to reduce moisture stress. A foliar spray may help increase calcium.

### *Tomato cuttings*

Let a branch sprawl on the ground. When it roots, cut it out and plant it somewhere else for a follow-on tomato crop. You can also cut a branch (the lower the better) and plant it about two thirds deep. Keep it moist and in semi-shade till it starts to grow. This is a good way to get a follow-on crop. It's also a good way to avoid ever buying tomato plants or seeds – just borrow a bit of someone else's.

### *Grafted tomatoes*

These can grow enormous and, in temperate areas, will fruit again the following year. Unfortunately many of the grafts are poor and you'll get either masses of leaves and no fruit, or the poor yellowy red small fruit of the graft. Watch your grafted tomato carefully and take off any branch that starts to bear tiny fruit. Probably nineteen out of twenty grafted tomato plants get taken over by shoots from below the graft.

The massive plants may also produce only a few tomatoes till late in the season. Even though they'll survive till next year you may still be better off with an early annual tomato planted in spring – but you will save the effort of having to plant them again.

Tomatoes can be grafted onto potatoes. This is fun, though you get slightly fewer tomatoes and potatoes than you would otherwise have. Tomatoes can also be grafted onto native solanums like kangaroo berry. This gives very frost resistant plants, but the grafts often fail and it can be difficult to get kangaroo berry plants ... and you don't get much fruit anyway.

### *Other 'perennial' tomatoes*

Tomatoes are potentially perennial in frost free climates, but are usually grown as annuals as they die from wilts and other diseases before the end of their first season. Young tomatoes are much more wilt and virus resistant.

### *Keeping tomatoes over winter in cool climates*

Our worst frost was minus 8°C this year (usually it's only minus 5°C), but I was still picking two large tomatoes a week from an outside bush and a cup full of cherry tomatoes. It wasn't worth it. The tomatoes were a nice red colour but tasteless, almost bitter. I should have grated beetroot into our salads for colour instead, and relied on bottled or dried tomatoes for cooking.

How did I do it? I built a walled garden (or rather Bryan did) – stone terraces facing the morning sun with heat absorbing paving stones below and the warmth of the house nearby to reflect heat too. The top terraces were the warmest. I crowded the tomato plants with cauliflowers to insulate them and kept the soil below covered in calendulas to trap heat too.

The tomato plants were still growing in spring.

Another tomato that survived the winter was a climbing yellow tomato, wandering up and around an old spreading tamarillo. The tamarillo insulated it, at least till it got frosted off too (it regrew), but the yellow tomatoes had no more flavour than the others.

I find cherry tomatoes are the most frost resistant, especially if buried in the rest of the garden's jungle. Grafted tomatoes also tolerate cold, and except in very cold areas may sprout again the next year. Tomatoes planted in late summer survive early frost better than the tired old ones from spring.

You can also graft your own tomatoes onto native frost resistant stock like kangaroo berry. The trouble is that kangaroo berry isn't a prolific grower – and you'll get very few tomatoes in either summer or winter. But if you are keen on winter tomatoes you could try it – or build a glasshouse instead.

A simpler solution is to dig up your tomatoes in autumn and pot them – or grow new ones in pots, planted in late summer so they are in full vigour for winter. Keep them indoors at night and put them out in the sun during the day. They will be sweeter than my outdoor winter tomatoes – but still not as sweet as the ones that get the summer sun.

Grafted tomatoes can become short-lived perennials in warm climates or if you grow them against a warm north-facing wall in cooler climates – or grow them in a pot and take them indoors at night in winter.

### *Potted tomatoes*

Tomatoes do well in pots – it's a good way to get early tomatoes in spring or keep tomatoes fruiting through winter. The bigger the pot the better. You can even grow them on the window sill if you have a big window enclosure – or you prune your tomato bush every couple of days. Potted tomatoes can be kept out of frost reach, and will crop through winter.

Feed often – there won't be enough nutrients in the pot to give you a decent crop.

### ***Other ways to grow tomatoes***

*Tomatoes in a pile of tyres*

This is a good method for cold areas. The tyres are high and out of reach of mild frosts and the black absorbs heat.

Make piles of tyres two or three high. If three high, drive a stake down the middle so they are stable.

Fill with soil, then top with compost or good potting mix – or just feed extra well. Plant your tomatoes. They'll sprawl down the sides of the tyre pile. You'll get a crop 2 to 6 weeks earlier – and be safe from at least mild late frosts.

*Tomatoes in drainage pipe*

This is similar to the above method – but the ceramic pipes are prettier. I manage to get grafted tomatoes to stay healthy all winter in drainage pipes.

*Tomatoes under glass*

In very cold areas many gardeners simply grow tomatoes in a glass house – and in temperate areas they can be overwintered under glass. First find your glasshouse – or just make a temporary one with old windows balanced on a temporary wall of bricks.

## *COMPANION PLANTING WITH TOMATOES*

When grown together the scent of tomatoes appears to mask that of cabbages and vice versa – this helps repel the pests of both.

Tomatoes and eggplant appear to stunt each other. They are subject to a similar range of pests and diseases and have the same soil requirements. Possibly they simply compete on too many levels.

Don't grow tomatoes near stone fruit – both will attract fruit fly and may cross-infect. If possible, don't grow tomatoes in a block together. Scatter them through the garden to make it harder for fruit fly to find them.

If fusarium wilt is a problem, plant tomatoes after a thickly planted crop of broad beans – their root excretions will inhibit the fungus. The potash in comfrey or lucerne may help as may a companion crop of thickly planted garlic. Use the garlic tops as mulch. Practise crop rotation if fusarium wilt is expected.

## *GROWING PAINS*

Tomatoes are subject to various wilts and blotches. Some are transferred in seed. Others survive in the soil. If you had problems with tomatoes the year before, cover the soil with clear plastic for three weeks before you plant the next crop.

### *Fruit fly*

You'll find maggots in the fruit. Pick fruit regularly. Don't let fallen fruit lie on the ground. As a last resort, pick green tomatoes and let them ripen indoors or cover them with a fruit fly proof net made of old nylon stocking with a wire support. You can also put out fruit fly traps – old fruit juice with a pinch of yeast in a trap made from an old soft drink bottle with the top cut off, then inverted to make a funnel. You need at least one trap for every four plants. Check often to make sure they are still fermenting. If they are not, replace the bait. See Companion planting for tomatoes.

### *Mites*

These are small insects under leaves, causing mottled, dehydrated leaves – especially bad in dry weather or in glasshouses. Water under the leaves as well as on top.

### *Split fruit*

Uneven watering – too dry then very wet. Mulch, mulch and mulch.

### *Slugs and snails*

These are less of a problem for tomatoes than other veg, though they will eat your nice ripe tomatoes. Put a sharp collar made from the top of a can around the stem, or put pellets inside an old icecream container with a little door cut out for the snails, etc. to enter. This way the pellets won't kill worms and other soil life – or kids, dogs, cats and lizards.

### *Birds*

Pick fruit often. Use bird nets.

***Blossom end rot***

Blossom end rot shows as a dark patch on the fruit. It is due to irregular watering or lack of calcium. Mulch well to reduce water stress. A calcium foliar spray will increase calcium, a seaweed, compost, nettle or other 'green' spray every few days will also help. A half strength bordeaux spray can also be used, but as bordeaux will kill predators as well as help the blossom rot, try to cure the calcium deficiency first. If your soil is calcium deficient you may need to add dolomite to the garden generally or bring in materials for mulch and compost from areas that aren't calcium deficient.

***Cracked tomatoes***

This results from fluctuating moisture levels. Thick mulch and well drained soil will help prevent it. Don't let tomatoes dry out between waterings. Don't saturate them either. Lots of organic matter in the soil from frequently renewed mulch helps regulate moisture levels.

***Cutworms***

Plants appear suddenly cut off at the base. Try collars of old tin cans, old plastic soft drink bottles or stiff cardboard or two toothpicks as stakes on either side of seedlings. Try a green manure crop of mustard before planting. A well mulched soil will deter cutworms.

***Damping off***

Seedlings suddenly die; a brownish band may appear at ground level.

Dip seedlings in chamomile tea before planting, pour the rest around each one on planting. Make sure all organic matter in the soil is decomposed and no mulch is actually touching the seedlings.

***Red spider mites***

Webbed or dehydrated leaves.

A good solid overhead watering every day may be all this problem needs. In bad cases that don't respond to this use any of the repellent sprays or, as a last resort, spray tops and undersides of the leaves with white oil if the temperature is less than 24°C, with soap spray in the evenings or with pyrethrum spray.

***Blotchy tomatoes***

Hard yellow patches on ripe or near ripe tomatoes are usually caused by phosphorus or potash deficiency. Try a foliar tea made with potash or phosphorus rich materials – compost, seaweed, hen manure, comfrey, urine or use a potash or phosphorus rich fertiliser.

*Root knot nematodes*

Unthrifty plants that fail to thrive.

Mulch well to encourage earthworms – these are the best possible destroyers of nematodes, as well as the fungal webs of decomposing organic matter – the nematodes get caught and die. Grow marigolds (Tagetes spp) *close* around the plants. Marigolds deter root knot nematode (but not some other problem species), but if they are grown too far away the nematodes will be deterred – away from the marigolds and towards the tomatoes.

***Fusarium wilt***

With fusarium wilt the whole plant wilts, rotted at the base of the stem and stems may be cracked. In mild cases the plant may just grow slowly or be pale and stunted.

Fusarium wilt is a soil borne fungus. Try covering the soil before you plant out tomatoes with clear plastic sheeting for three weeks to kill off spores in the soil. Practice crop rotation and use resistant cultivars.

As soon as symptoms appear try double strength garlic spray on stems, soil and foliage. Seedlings can be dipped in garlic spray before planting out, with a little drizzled onto nearby soil. Soils high in potash are more resistant to fusarium wilt. Try adding wood ash or compost. In bad cases dig out plants and burn them. The spores are both wind and soil borne and will easily spread to neighbouring plants. Cover the hole with clear plastic or drench the soil in double strength garlic spray – or both. See companion planting for tomatoes.

***Small holes in fruit***

This is caused by tomato fruit worm. Don't worry about them – the damage usually isn't severe enough to worry about unless you are growing them commercially. As a last resort use DIPEL – a form of bacterial warfare on caterpillars, but harmless to other species.

***Poor fruit set***

This may be caused by too much nitrogen, particularly if foliage is thick and green – use mulch, compost, etc. (see under Feeding, p. 151). Try adding ground rock phosphate as a temporary measure. Some tomato varieties don't set well in cool weather, cold climate varieties may not set in very hot weather.

***Misshapen fruit***

Poor pollination, possibly caused by very hot or very cold weather. Possibly also a virus.

***'Rolled over' older leaves***

This can occur when you have hot days and cold nights. Don't worry about it. It's not a virus.

***Yellow leaves***

Yellow older leaves means nitrogen deficiency – feed more. Yellowing between leaves may be magnesium or potash deficiency. Add wood ash, comfrey mulch. See also 'Feeding tomatoes'.

## *FROM THE GARDEN TO THE TABLE*

***Harvesting tomatoes***

*Fresh eating period* Frost free period minus about 16 weeks for early maturers. Tomatoes can be grown inside in pots in winter; tomato bushes with unripened fruit should be hung in a sheltered spot to continue ripening over the next month. Most green tomatoes will gradually ripen indoors. You may get tomatoes all year round with the last two methods.

*Storage time* Several weeks in fridge. Green tomatoes may keep for months.

*Food value* 88 kj per 10 g. Excellent source of vitamin C, also A and potassium.

Be prepared to become a home-grown tomato addict. Nothing tastes like a fresh tomato – certainly not the pink golf balls you find in supermarkets. These travel well and slice neatly. A good tomato hardly slices at all – it oozes bright red juice.

The riper and redder a tomato when you pick it, the sweeter it'll be. Tomatoes do ripen after they're picked however – even dark green ones will slowly ripen indoors in winter.

In fruit fly prone areas it's best to pick tomatoes when they are just starting to colour – the faintest blush of pink – and make sure *every* fallen one is picked up.

*Ripening green tomatoes*

If your bush is too big to dig up and pot, pull it up by the roots and leave it in the shed. The tomatoes will keep ripening as the stems keep feeding them.

Pick green tomatoes before they are damaged by frost. Store them on newspaper inside. They'll keep ripening for months – and the flavour will still be much better than shop ones. Just spread the tomatoes on newspaper (to soak up the juice if any go rotten) in a warm room. Inspect them every few days and toss out bad ones. They won't be as sweet as the ones you picked at the height of summer, but will have more flavour than shop-bought tomatoes.

You can also cook green tomatoes. They make good sauce, chutney, etc.

### *How to peel a tomato*

Cut just through the skin, no deeper, from top to bottom and back again, so you've divided the tomato into quarters. Now pour boiling (or just very hot) water over the tomato for a few seconds. The edges of the cuts will peel back and you can peel the rest of the skin off.

Peeled tomatoes are much nicer sliced on sandwiches and infinitely better in soup and stews unless they are going to be puréed – otherwise you end up with wrinkly bits at the bottom.

## *Dealing with surplus tomatoes*

Simple 10 minute preserved tomatoes

Take ripe, firm small tomatoes. They must have no bruise or blemish at all. Make sure they are clean and quite dry.

Place them in a tall, deep jar, one at a time – again, make sure they do not squash, bruise or split. Cover with oil right to the top of the jar. Seal. Keep in the fridge till needed. These will keep up to six months or even longer.

*TOMATOES AND ONIONS*

If you are cooking tomatoes with onions, sauté the onions till they are soft before adding the tomatoes, otherwise the onions will stay tough and not melt away.

*TOMATO PASTE*

There are dozens of ways of making tomato paste. Try chopping the tomatoes, add no water and simmer till they are thick and bubbling like magma – great bursts of bubbles that spread over the kitchen. Spread the mixture on alfoil and leave in the sun till dry – take indoors in wet weather or at night. Now roll the sticky mixture into balls, dip each ball in a cup of oil and store in sealed glass jars in the frig. Take out a ball as you need it. Otherwise just stuff the paste in a jar and cover the lot with oil – though this can give an uneven surface as you use it which may not be oil covered, so you can lose some of the paste to fungus.

If you don't want to dry the paste in the sun boil it down as far as possible with a tablespoon of white vinegar or half a teaspoon of citric acid for every four cups of tomatoes. Pack the thick purée into glass jars, cover with a film of oil. Place the jars in the oven in a tray of water and cook till the water just boils. Leave till cool and seal.

The paste can be flavoured at the simmering stage with garlic, black pepper or very finely chopped basil or thyme.

*TOMATO SAUCE*

6 kilos tomatoes (red or green – add more sugar if green)
1 litre white vinegar
1 kilo chopped onions, sautéed till soft in a little oil

150 grams sugar
10 cloves chopped garlic
teaspoon ground ginger
pepper and salt to taste

Boil for two hours, strain through a sieve. Bottle. A little melted clarified butter or lard (the traditional sealer) on top before sealing will help it to keep longer and keep the colour brighter.

*CLASSIC TOMATO SALAD*

Slice very red ripe tomatoes. Douse with good olive oil. Serve at once.

A few torn basil leaves or a little chopped garlic may be added. Ripe tomatoes are both sweet and acid and shouldn't need anything else.

*DRIED TOMATOES*

Home dried tomatoes still taste of the sun.

Halve or quarter your tomatoes, spread them in the sun on alfoil on a very hot day. Take them in at night. They should be dry in about three days, depending on the amount of sunlight.

Layer them in a jar and cover with olive oil. You can add fresh basil and garlic to the oil to taste.

I add dried tomatoes:

- roughly chopped to winter salads.
- whole with artichokes, potatoes and mayonnaise.
- with camembert and lettuce and vinaigrette dressing.
- cooked in a about a hundred ways.

*TOMATO SANDWICHES*

The secret here is to butter evenly, thickly and everywhere so the juice doesn't soften the bread – or use cheese to protect the bread instead.

Crackers and cheese with a thick slice of ripe tomato are one of life's delicacies – with a good grind of black pepper.

*TOMATOES AND GOOD BREAD*

Take a thick slice of fresh French or Italian bread. Brush olive oil on both sides. Toast lightly on both sides, top with fresh tomato, with or without bocconcino cheese and lots of torn basil leaves or a thick spread of pesto and thinly sliced very ripe tomato or eggplant in olive oil with a thin slice of fresh tomato – the possibilities are endless . . .

*TOMATOES IN CREAM*

Pour a cup of cream into a pan with four cloves of chopped garlic. Simmer for ten minutes. Cut four very ripe peeled tomatoes in half and lay them in the cream. Cook gently till they are heated through. Take off the heat before they turn soggy and top with finely chopped parsley, basil or fresh coriander.

*SIMPLE PASTA SAUCE*

Sauté two onions and 12 cloves of garlic in olive oil till soft. Add 12 peeled chopped tomatoes. Cook till soft. Add a lot of chopped basil, chives, parsley – or marjoram or oregano instead.

This isn't as garlicky as it seems, as the garlic is cooked in oil first and loses most of its pungency.

Scatter cheese on top – parmesan or pecorino or even mozzarella – grind on black pepper at the last minute – it goes bitter if you add it too soon.

# *seed sources*

These all supply excellent mail order catalogues and growing instructions.

***Diggers Club Seeds***
'Heronswood', 105 Latrobe Parade, Dromana, Victoria 3936
Excellent mail order seed catalogue, often superb range of varieties, often heirloom and difficult to obtain or specialist seeds, e.g. capsicums specifically for cooking or tomatoes for drying.

***Phoenix Seeds***
PO Box 9, Stanley, Tasmania 7331
Specialises in open pollinated (non-hybrid) varieties.

***Eden Seeds***
MS 316, Gympie, Queensland 4570.
A family-operated company specialising in open pollinated, non-hybrid seeds.

***The Seed Savers Network***
Box 975, Byron Bay, NSW 2481
An essential organisation for anyone who wants to grow – or save – rare or special plants. Run by Michel and Jude Fanton (who produce the excellent *Seed Saver's Handbook*) you will receive a biannual newsletter with offers of seed and plant swapping, biodiversity news, permaculture advice, and a lot more.

# *other books*

***BY JACKIE FRENCH***

***A-Z of Useful Plants***
*Recommended Retail Price* **$14.95**

***Backyard Self-sufficiency***
*Recommended Retail Price* **$14.95**

***Household Self-sufficiency***
*Recommended Retail Price* **$16.95**

***Jackie French's Guide to Companion Planting***
*Recommended Retail Price* **$9.95**

***Natural Control of Garden Pests***
*Recommended Retail Price* **$15.95**

***New Plants from Old***
Simple, natural, no-cost plant propagation
*Recommended Retail Price* **$16.95**

***Organic Control of Household Pests***
New, completely revised edition
*Recommended Retail Price* **$13.95**

***Organic Control of Common Weeds***
*Recommended Retail Price* **$13.95**

***Soil Food***
1372 ways to add fertility to your soil
*Recommended Retail Price* **$16.95**

***Switch!***
Home-based power, water and sewerage systems for the 21st century
*Recommended Retail Price* **$17.95**

***The Wilderness Garden***
Beyond Organic Gardening
*Recommended Retail Price* **$19.95**